Men'sHealth.
TRAINING
LOG

Track Your Workouts to
Build Your Best Body Ever

By the Editors of Men's Health

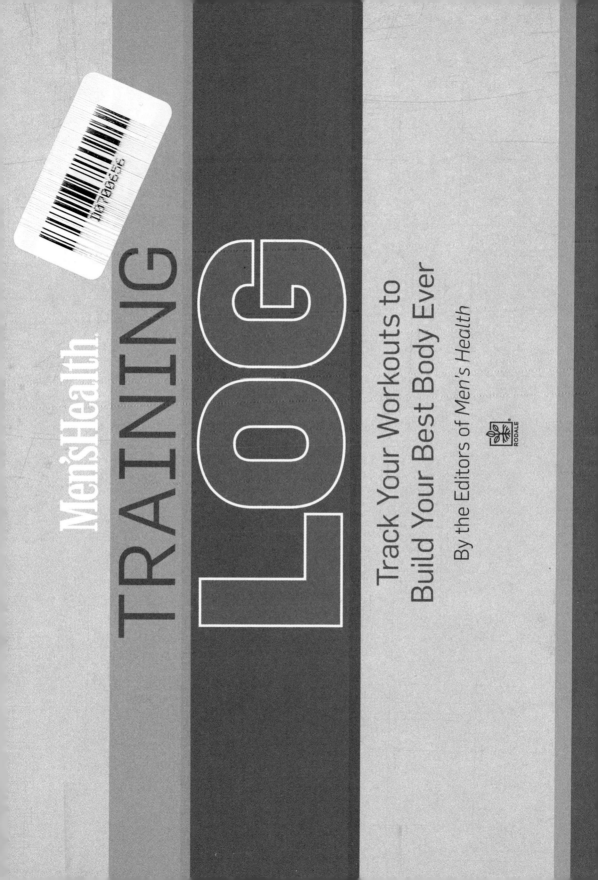

RODALE

Notice

The information in this book is meant to supplement, not replace, proper exercise training. All forms of exercise pose some inherent risks. The editors and publisher advise readers to take full responsibility for their safety and know their limits. Before practicing the exercises in this book, be sure that your equipment is well maintained, and do not take risks beyond your level of experience, aptitude, training, and fitness. The exercise and dietary programs in this book are not intended as a substitute for any exercise routine or dietary regimen that may have been prescribed by your doctor. As with all exercise and dietary programs, you should get your doctor's approval before beginning.

Mention of specific companies, organizations, or authorities in this book does not imply endorsement by the author or publisher, nor does mention of specific companies, organizations, or authorities imply that they endorse this book, its author, or the publisher.

Internet addresses and telephone numbers given in this book were accurate at the time it went to press.

© 2007 by Rodale Inc.

All rights reserved. No part of this publication may be reproduced or transmitted in any form or by any means, electronic or mechanical, including photocopying, recording, or any other information storage and retrieval system, without the written permission of the publisher.

Rodale books may be purchased for business or promotional use or for special sales. For information, please write to:

Special Markets Department, Rodale Inc., 733 Third Avenue, New York, NY 10017

Men's Health® is a registered trademark of Rodale Inc.

Printed in the United States of America

Rodale Inc. makes every effort to use acid-free ⊗, recycled paper ♻.

Library of Congress Cataloging-in-Publication Data

ISBN 13: 978-1-59486-666-1
ISBN 10: 1-59486-666-X

Distributed to the trade by Macmillan

2 4 6 8 10 9 7 5 3 1 paperback

RODALE
LIVE YOUR WHOLE LIFE™

We inspire and enable people to improve their lives and the world around them

For more of our products visit **rodalestore.com** or call 800-848-4735

Men'sHealth.
If you want to build muscle, improve your sex life,
and do nearly everything better, visit our Web site at
menshealth.com

CONTENTS

HOW TO USE THIS LOG

The *Men's Health Training Log* provides the perfect framework to help you keep track of your workouts—whether you're seeking weight loss, muscle gain, or you're just looking to chart your progress in the gym.

This is your own personal training log, so there is no right or wrong way to use it. You may use this training log to plan your strength-training and cardiovascular workouts, and to record the activities and exercises you've completed. Use it as a way to chart what you've done both in and out of the gym, as well as to record what you enjoyed most, what worked, and what didn't work. To keep you motivated and informed, the log is filled with the same top-notch advice from the pros that is featured in *Men's Health* magazine, including tips or nutrition, effective weight training, and cardiovascular workouts. If you're already a seasoned veteran of the gym, use the advice to supplement or fine-tune the workout you're already doing—for even better, faster results. On the other hand, if you'd consider yourself a gym newbie—or it's been so long since your last workout that that's how you feel—use the three-step fitness plan beginning on page 6 as a starting point to seeing results in just 5 weeks.

This log can act as a friend, motivator, and coach. It will serve as a constant reminder of where you want to be fitness-wise and how you plan to get there. For best results, carry your log with you at all times. Pull it out when you need extra motivation to exercise, or when you are tempted to skip the gym and instead swing by a fast-food restaurant for a burger on the way home.

Speaking of motivation, nothing is more likely to keep you showing up for your workouts than seeing results—in the form of a stronger, more flexible body that is better able to take you the distance. That's why before you do anything, we want you to take a couple of minutes to write down a few benchmarks of your fitness levels today—so that later, you can see just how far you've come.

MEASURE YOUR SUCCESS

Before you start, use the following fitness tests to gauge your current levels of strength, flexibility, and endurance. After 5 weeks, repeat the assessments. "You can expect improvements of 15 to 20 percent across the board," says Mike Mejia, CSCS, MS, coauthor of *Scrawny to Brawny* and author of *Men's Health Better Body Blueprint*. As for muscle gain and fat loss, the following plan works for both. Snap a digital photo now and another after 35 days, and your new body image will be all the proof you'll need.

Test your strength. Do as many classic pushups as you can without stopping, but use this precise execution: Take 2 seconds to lower your body until your upper arms dip below your elbows; pause for 1 second; then take 1 second to push your body up. This ensures that you'll perform the test identically each time you take it.

Test your flexibility. Place a yardstick on the floor and put a foot-long piece of masking tape across the 15-inch mark. Sit down with your legs out in front of you and your heels at the edge of the tape, one on each side of the yardstick. Put one hand on top of the other and reach forward over the yardstick as far as you can by bending at your hips. The number your fingertips touch is your benchmark.

Test your endurance. On a treadmill or on a flat course outdoors, run or walk 1.5 miles as fast as you can, and record your time. (Warm up first by walking or jogging at an easy pace for 5 minutes.)

THE THREE-STEP FITNESS PLAN

If it's been longer than you care to remember—or admit out loud—since you last worked out seriously, the following three-step fitness plan is for you. It's backed by science but built around your life—to conquer your time constraints, speed your progress, and simplify your workouts.

It's designed to increase muscle size and strength, improve flexibility and endurance, and, of course, burn fat—all in less than 90 minutes a week. Start now and you're the odds-on favorite to be fit in 5 weeks.

STEP 1: ADOPT A 3-DAY STANDARD

In a recent survey, the National Center for Health Statistics found that only 19 percent of Americans do three or more intense workouts a week. Given these hard numbers, it's unrealistic to expect that you'll suddenly start exercising for 6 or 7 days straight. Fortunately, that level of commitment isn't necessary. "You'll see most of the benefits of exercise by working out hard just three times a week," says Mejia. "And that's especially true if you're out of shape." Use these strategies to make sure you stick to the plan.

Save one workout for the weekend. "Even if Saturday and Sunday are packed with family commitments and various home-improvement projects, it's likely that you'll still have more free time then than on any given weekday," says John Raglin, PhD, an exercise psychologist at Indiana University in Bloomington. And that means you'll have to fit in only two sessions between Monday and Friday.

Track the ancillary benefits. Keep a job-performance journal on the days you exercise and the days you don't exercise. Each day, rate these three categories on a scale of 1 (poor) to 7 (excellent).

1. Your ability to work without stopping to take unscheduled breaks
2. Your ability to stick to your routine or plan (your "to do" list) for the day
3. Your overall job performance

"It's likely you'll find that you score higher and do more on the days you exercise, despite taking time out for your workout," says Jim McKenna, PhD, professor of physical activity and health at Leeds Metropolitan University, in the United Kingdom. (Make sure you compare days that are similar in workload.) And this will reinforce your motivation to keep at it.

Keep your streak intact. Research shows that when men skip a workout, there's a 62 percent chance they'll miss an exercise session the following week. Worse, "a single lapse can result in feelings of failure that are so overwhelming, a person will just quit, even though he successfully followed through with exercise 99 percent of the time," says Dr. Raglin. Institute this policy: If you don't have time for your entire workout, take 10 minutes and do a port on of your routine—even if it's only a couple of sets of pushups and lunges.

STEP 2: GO HARD, NOT LONG

Cap your exercise sessions at 30 minutes. YMCA researchers found that men were twice as likely to stick to an exercise program when they did shorter workouts—30 minutes or less—than when they did longer sessions. "They also gained more muscle and lost more fat, because they worked at a higher intensity, instead of just going through the motions of a long workout," says Wayne Westcott, CSCS, PhD, coauthor of the study. Here's how to streamline your routine.

Work every muscle, every workout. University of Alabama researchers found that men who trained their entire bodies each session, 3 days a week, gained 10 pounds of muscle in 3 months. In fact, they packed on four times more muscle than, and lost twice as much fat as, men who worked each muscle group only once a week. It doesn't take a lot; the big gainers did just nine total sets in each session, about the same as two sets each of five exercises.

Use a modified circuit routine. Do one set of each exercise in a consecutive fashion, but—unlike with a classic circuit—rest after each. "You'll improve recovery between sets, which will allow you to give your best effort each time, the key to optimal gains," says Bill Hartman CSCS, PT, a strength coach and physical therapist in Indianapolis. Why the circuit approach? Your rest periods will be shorter than if you performed back-to-back sets of the same exercise—so you'll save time.

Use this simple trick to gauge the ideal downtime: "Rest between exercises only as long as it takes for your breathing rate to return to normal," says Hartman. As you become better conditioned, you'll automatically take less time between sets. This ensures that your workout is as challenging in week 5 as it was in week 1.

Finish with cardio. After your weight session, dedicate the remainder of your time to running, cycling, or rowing. Don't worry about the clock: "You'll improve your conditioning more by running at a high intensity for 15 minutes than with the slow 30-minute jog that most guys do," says Mejia.

STEP 3: KEEP IT SIMPLE

Forget about target heart rates and three-digit lifting tempos. "Working out isn't rocket science," says Mejia. "You just need to challenge your body a little bit more each session." The keys to doing just that, without thinking twice:

Trust your lungs. In a recent study at the University of Wisconsin at Lacrosse, researchers discovered that running at a pace that allows you to talk—but only in short spurts of three or four words at a time—is approximately the same as exercising at your

"ventilatory threshold," or the highest intensity you can sustain for the duration of your cardio session. By gauging your effort this way, you exercise as hard as possible without running out of gas too early.

Trust your judgment. "Without counting, lower the weight slowly and lift it fast," says Mejia. George Washington University researchers showed that lifters who used this technique gained two times more strength than those who performed each repetition at a slow speed from start to finish. Don't worry about taking an exact amount of time: Just think "slow" or "fast" as you move the weight; your body will react accordingly.

Trust your muscles. In general, use the heaviest weight that allows you to perform all your repetitions without reaching failure. One caveat: Instead of defining "failure" as the point at which you can't complete one more repetition ("absolute failure"), employ the concept of "technical failure," says Hartman. That's the point at which your body posture changes—you have to cheat by leaning forward or back to complete the movement—or you can't control the speed of the weight you're lifting. For instance, if the rate at which you perform a pushup starts to slow as you press yourself to the starting position, you've achieved technical failure. Consider that the end of your set. The reason: Once you've hit technical failure, fewer target muscle fibers are firing during each repetition thereafter—so you've achieved maximal benefit from that exercise.

START TODAY

Write down your primary goal. Be specific: Whether you want to lose 20 pounds of fat, gain 10 pounds of muscle, or complete your first triathlon, give yourself one major objective and put it on paper. (For more on creating clear fitness goals, including short-term goals to guide you every step of the way as you work toward your primary goal, see "Setting Goals" on page 10.) Schedule your first three workouts. Plan the date, time, and place of each session in Outlook or your day planner. You'll be less likely to allow meetings or social events to interfere with your workouts. Be sure to block off a big-enough chunk to account for any time needed to change your clothes, shower, or travel to the gym—the forgotten factors that doom workouts. Use this workout log. This will give you tangible numbers to improve on with each workout.

When you've reached your goal—when you've transformed yourself from Out-of-Shape Guy to a leaner, more muscular, more fit version of your former self—that's just the beginning. Use the dozens of ideas and tips you'll find scattered throughout this training log to ratchet up your workout for even greater returns on your investment. (They're also great ways to overcome a training plateau, where your body has

become so adept at performing your current workout program that you no longer see improvement in muscle size, strength, or weight loss.) Make a new goal and attack it with the same determination you used to meet the first one, but this time perhaps step it up to four or five workouts a week, add a new cardio exercise such as cycling or rowing, or add some variations on the classics to your weight-lifting routine, such as replacing your traditional bench press with a dumbbell twisting bench press or doing a few Swiss-ball pushups instead of the usual version. Just be sure to write it all down in your training log, so that you can see how far you've come—and exactly what you need to do to keep on reaching your goals.

WRITE OFF YOUR BELLY

When it comes to losing your gut, perhaps the details don't matter. People who keep a basic food journal lose as much weight as those who record every single bite, report University of Pittsburgh researchers. In the recent study, scientists found that dieters who simply wrote down the size of each meal (small, medium, large, XL) were just as successful at losing weight as those who tracked the specific foods, calories, and fat they ate. "The process of simply keeping a food diary may be more important than the information you record," says study author Diane Helsel, RD. "It may serve as a reminder of how much you're eating over the course of a day."

Researchers project that watching television during dinner just two times a week will result in an 8-pound weight gain over the course of a year.

SETTING GOALS

As you embark on a year's worth of workouts, it's important to set goals. Clear fitness goals will give you something to work toward, keep you motivated, and provide you with a sense of purpose when you step into the weight room or onto the treadmill. For maximum success, make sure the goals you set are specific, attainable, realistic, and wide-ranging. Your goals should be tailored to your fitness level and capabilities, yet they should be lofty enough to force you to push yourself. Because you will be doing cardiovascular exercise as well as strength training, you should set specific goals within each category. And if you want to shed pounds, you should set weight-loss goals as well. For example, you may want to set a goal of losing 15 pounds through a combination of increased cardiovascular exercise and regular weight training. A more specific goal would be to do this by eating at least 25 grams of fiber and 5 to 10 fruits and vegetables per day. Because you set goals, plan for both the short and long term. Because they are more achievable, short-term goals help you gain a sense of

GREAT EXPECTATIONS

Most experts recommend setting modest weight-reduction goals, but a new study from the University of Minnesota suggests that having high weight-loss expectations may help you lose a greater amount of weight. The researchers found that men who tried to lose an average of 16 percent of their body weight—instead of the commonly recommended 5 to 10 percent—did indeed drop more than their conservative counterparts. "They seem to understand that it takes more effort to lose more weight," speculates Jennifer Linde, PhD, the lead researcher. Make your overall goal as lofty as you like—20, 30, or even 50 pounds—but set a practical time frame, capping expectations at an average loss of 1 pound a week.

accomplishment, and they give you a reason to celebrate as you work toward your long-term aspirations.

It is important, however, not to set too many goals at once. Try to keep your goals down to one or two long-term goals per category (strength training, cardiovascular exercise, and nutrition), and keep your short-term goals focused and to a minimum as well. And realize that your goals don't have to be set in stone; if you realize that a goal or strategy clearly isn't working, get rid of it and set a new one. In order to be successful in your exercise plan, you have to remain flexible.

As you complete your short-term goals, always think a few steps ahead. In other words, before you reach the goal you are striving for, plan out goals for the following few months or weeks (depending on the goals), so you constantly keep your eye on the prize: a fitter, healthier, and slimmer you.

One great way to stick to the goals you've set is to have a training partner, someone who will get you off the couch and into the gym, even when you are having an off day—someone who will make you feel good about yourself on the days you feel your goals are out of reach.

FIVE EASY RULES TO REVEAL YOUR MUSCLE

You love lifting. You love the plain challenge and the simple rewards—beating your previous best and feeling a great pump afterward. But if gaining mass is all you focus on, soon no one will be able to distinguish your traps from your deltoids. For a lean and chiseled physique, you need cardio work. Relax—no distance running involved.

Besides, you know you need aerobic exercise for a healthy heart. And a healthy heart is more efficient at transporting blood and oxygen to working muscles. The stronger your heart, the stronger each of its contractions. That means more oxygenated blood is pumped out with each beat.

What follows is a set of rules to help lifters build healthy hearts. You don't need much cardio work, and most of what you do need should be done at high intensity, as befits a man with a lifter's mindset. It'll help you see more muscle definition without wasting time in the gym spinning your wheels.

RULE 1: CHANGE THE CYCLE

You don't lift the same way all year, so why should the frequency, intensity, and duration of your cardiovascular workouts stay the same? They shouldn't.

When you're trying to add muscle, keep your aerobic work to a minimum—say, once or twice a week for about 15 to 20 minutes. This will limit your energy expenditure and allow your body to concentrate on building muscle.

When you're trying to get lean, increase your cardio training to two to four times a week, to help strip away excess body fat.

At all times, alternate your cardio methods so your workout's not so boring—treadmill running one day, rowing or elliptical training the next, cycling the day after that.

RULE 2: SEPARATE CARDIO FROM LIFTING

Serious lifters worry that cardiovascular training will impede their ability to recover from intense strength training. That all depends on when and how you do your cardio.

Keep your cardio days and strength days as removed from each other as possible. That way, your cardio won't hinder gains in strength and size. For instance, doing a tough cycling workout after you hammer your legs with squats and lunges isn't a good idea if your goal is to build bigger legs. Save your cardio for the next day, or even 2 days later, to rest your legs.

If you must do cardio and weight training on the same day, choose a form of aerobic work that emphasizes body parts your weight lifting didn't focus on that day. So, if your cardio choice is rowing, which works your upper body as much as it does your legs, row on a day when your weight session doesn't concentrate on your upper-body muscles.

Whichever route you choose, just be sure to hit the weights first. You don't want to wipe yourself out before your weight routine—you won't get the most out of your session, and lifting when you're tired can be dangerous.

RULE 3: DON'T MAKE AN IMPACT

Your body has enough to contend with in repairing the damage that lifting inflicts on it. The last thing you need to do is break it down further with high-impact cardio training.

Concentrate on cardio workouts that minimize microtrauma—the small tears to muscle fibers that are part of the process of building new muscle. Running on hard surfaces like asphalt or concrete can be traumatic to muscles and joints. Jumping rope can cause similar problems. Your best bets for low-impact exercise are swimming, cycling, and using an elliptical machine.

RULE 4: IGNORE THE "FAT-BURNING ZONE"

It's a myth that you have to work out continuously for 20 minutes before you begin burning fat. The thinking once was that you needed to exercise in a range between 60 and 80 percent of your maximum heart rate. Any lower was too easy, and any higher made it too difficult to efficiently use fat for fuel.

Ignore that theory. Your body uses more energy overall when training at high intensities—just look at the physique of a sprinter. Going all out also makes better use of your time. You can finish your cardio in an intense 10- to 15-minute workout.

Stick to interval workouts that feature short bursts of high-intensity movement followed by active recovery periods. (See the following sample workouts.) This approach is best for your heart and for fat loss.

RULE 5: CHOOSE THE PATH OF MORE RESISTANCE

Changing the gears on a bike and altering the gradient on a treadmill, for instance, are great ways to increase intensity. Just be careful to find a level of resistance that won't reduce the amount of work you're able to do when you return to the weight room.

Now that you know the rules, follow these guidelines, depending on your goals.

BULK CYCLE (12 WEEKS)

Do this when you're trying to add muscle.

Frequency: Twice a week

Duration: 10 to 15 minutes (not including warmup and cooldown)

Protocol: Intervals

Intensity: High

Example: Stationary cycling

Warmup: 5 minutes of light pedaling

Work interval: 20 seconds of pedaling as fast as you can

Recovery interval: 40 seconds of light pedaling

Total reps: 10 to 15

Cooldown: 3 to 5 minutes of light pedaling

LEAN CYCLE (8 WEEKS)

Do this when you're trying to gain definition.

Frequency: Two to four times a week

Duration: 15 to 20 minutes (not including warmup and cooldown)

Protocol: Intervals

Intensity: High

Example: Rowing

Warmup: 3 to 5 minutes of light rowing

Work interval: 45 seconds of hard rowing

Recovery interval: 90 seconds easy

Total reps: 7 to 9

Cooldown: 3 to 5 minutes of light rowing

SIMPLIFY YOUR LIFTING PLAN, SUPERSIZE YOUR STRENGTH

It's important to know first that all of life's stressors, both physical and psychological, directly affect your performance in the gym—and they change from day to day. For instance, suppose you lift weights intensely on Monday after work, and then on Tuesday night you get only 5 hours of sleep, instead of your usual 7. Wednesday morning, your car's "check engine" light comes on as you pull in to work, and 5 minutes later your boss assigns you a high-priority project. When it's time for your evening workout, you aren't physically or mentally prepared to give your best effort.

And that means your strength and endurance will fade faster than in your previous workout. When this happens, it's a signal from your body that your muscles have had enough—that doing more repetitions won't lead to greater growth, but will only increase the stress on your body, slowing recovery time. There's a flip side, too: If your life has gone perfectly over the past couple of days, you may feel like you can lift the world. This is the time to take advantage of your increased ability—by upping weights, sets, and repetitions—in order to accelerate your muscle gains.

You see, your body provides the best indicator of how long your workout should last. And, chances are, you're doing more than you need—even on your best days. But use the four-step plan that follows and you'll never waste another repetition . . . or a minute in the gym that could be spent in the sun.

STEP 1: STREAMLINE YOUR WORKOUT

Although most men perform three or four exercises for each muscle group, it's better to choose just one. Fact is, you obtain almost all the size-boosting benefits of weight lifting from the first exercise you do, when your muscles are fresh. For example, let's say you complete three sets of each of these three chest exercises: flat bench press, incline bench press, and dumbbell fly. By the time you do the last exercise, the amount of weight you can handle is so low that it's no longer challenging enough to stimulate muscle growth.

Don't believe it? Try doing the exercises in reverse order. Not surprisingly, you'll be able to lift far less than usual for the flat bench press; you'll need to use a weight you'd normally consider too light. Which means there's no reason to think it's benefiting your muscles.

How to do it: You can apply this rule to your current workout—eliminating exercises that target the same muscle group—or use the 3-day-a-week plan below. It works your entire body with just four exercises each session.

Alternate between Workout A and Workout B every other day, doing the exercises in the order shown, and use this repetition strategy: The first time you perform Workout A, do six repetitions of each exercise; the next time, do 12 repetitions. In Workout B, do the opposite: 12 repetitions in the first session, six in the next. Continue to alternate for each workout. This ensures that you train your muscles for both muscular strength and muscular endurance, a method that leads to the fastest gains. As for the number of sets you'll perform, keep reading.

Workout A

1. Squat
2. Bench press
3. Bent-over row
4. Reverse crunch

Workout B

1. Deadlift
2. Chinup
3. Lateral raise
4. Side bridge

WORKOUT A

1. SQUAT

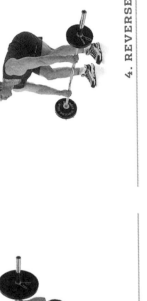

2. BENCH PRESS

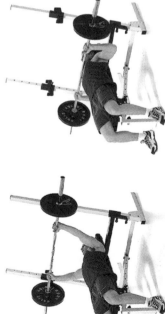

3. BENT-OVER ROW

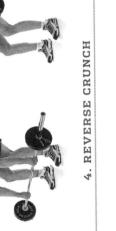

4. REVERSE CRUNCH

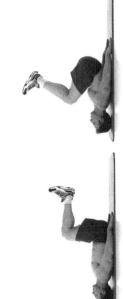

WORKOUT B

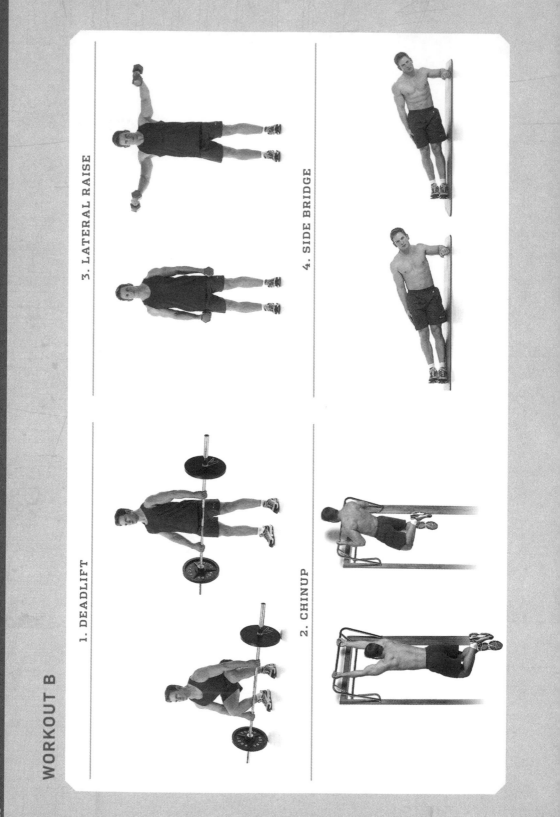

1. DEADLIFT

2. CHINUP

3. LATERAL RAISE

4. SIDE BRIDGE

STEP 2: REV UP YOUR ENGINE

Like Tiger Woods after blowing a third-round lead, your muscles perform better when they're fired up. So prime them for action by using a technique called the ramp-up method. By exciting the nerve pathways between your brain and muscles—without causing fatigue—it allows you to activate a greater number of muscle fibers than if you didn't warm up. The result: You'll be able to lift heavier weights and do more repetitions. And that means faster gains in both size and strength.

How to do it: For each exercise, estimate the weight you plan to use in your regular sets. (It doesn't have to be exact; just go with your best guess.) That's your base weight. Then perform the 2-minute warmup that follows. There's no need to rest between sets just change the weight and repeat. Once you've finished all three warmup sets, you're ready to start your regular sets.

Set 1: Five repetitions with 60 percent of your base weight.

Set 2: Three repetitions with 80 percent of your base weight.

Set 3: One repetition with 110 percent of your base weight. (By using a slightly heavier weight than your base on your last warmup set, you'll trick your brain into engaging even more muscle fibers during your regular sets.)

STEP 3: DETERMINE THE BEST WEIGHT

Here's where it gets fun: After you warm up (step 2), you'll test your strength to determine the ideal weight to use for your regular sets, using the benchmark of technical failure. Technical failure is the point at which your performance starts to decline, and it can be identified in two ways.

1. You can't maintain perfect form. The easiest gauge is when your posture changes—for instance, you have to arch your back to complete a bench press, or you need to lean your torso backward to complete an arm curl.

2. You aren't in total control of the weight. In this case, the speed at which you lift a weight slows down as you pass your "sticking point." The other yardstick: You aren't able to lower a weight back to the starting position at the same rate from top to bottom. That is, it feels as though the weight overtakes you.

When either of these conditions occurs, you've reached technical failure. Unlike in absolute failure, in which you can't perform even one more repetition, you'll probably feel as if you could pump out a couple more.

How to do it: For each exercise, start by estimating the amount of weight you think will allow you to complete your planned number of repetitions for that day. Don't worry if you're not sure; that's what the test is for. (Keep in mind this isn't a one-time assessment; you'll repeat the test for each exercise, every single workout.) Now do as many repetitions as you can, ending the set when you reach technical failure.

If you're able to complete all your planned repetitions—but no more—without achieving technical failure, you've chosen the correct weight. For example, if your goal was six repetitions, you would have achieved technical failure on repetition seven.

However, if you reach technical failure before you complete all your intended repetitions, the weight is too heavy. And if you're able to complete more reps than you planned, the weight is too light. In either case, rest for a minute or so, adjust the weight accordingly (up or down), and then repeat the test. It may take you a couple of tries to find the ideal weight, but that's okay: you're not wasting time, because you're still challenging your muscles.

STEP 4: LIFT TILL YOU DROP

The rest is simple: Once you've used technical failure to determine the ideal weight to use for an exercise, you'll simply perform as many

sets with that weight as you can—stopping when your performance drops off significantly. This is your cue that you've worked the target muscles maximally.

How to do it: Using the ideal weight (step 3), perform one set to technical failure. Next, rest as long as it takes for your breathing rate to return to normal (but no longer than 2 minutes). Then repeat the process as many times as you can, stopping when the number of repetitions you can complete is three lower than the number you planned. This is known as your performance drop-off. Consider this a signal from your body that it's time to move on to the next exercise in your workout (or to the locker room). So if your goal is six repetitions, you'll have performed your last set of that movement when you can't complete four repetitions without achieving technical failure. If your goal is 12 reps, the critical number is 10. You may be able to perform eight sets, six sets, or perhaps only one or two. Regardless, you can be sure that it's precisely the number your muscles need.

IS YOUR WORKOUT PAST ITS SELL-BY DATE?

In a hospital, using outdated information is considered malpractice; in a gym, it's standard operating procedure. Don't believe it? Take a look at today's most sacred lifting guidelines, and you'll find that some originated in the 1940s and '50s, a time when castration was a cutting-edge treatment for prostate cancer, and endurance exercise was thought to be harmful to women. What's worse, other, more recent recommendations regarding exercise form have been negated by new research, yet are still commonly prescribed by fitness professionals.

Chances are, these are the same rules you lift by right now. And that means your workout is long past due for a 21st-century overhaul. Keep in mind, I'm not suggesting that your current plan doesn't work. After all, at its most basic level, building muscle is simple: Pick up a heavy weight, put it down, repeat. But improve the details and avoid mistakes, and you'll build more muscle in less time, with less risk of injury. Put a check next to today's date—it marks the official expiration of your old workout.

THE AGE-OLD ADVICE: "DO 8 TO 12 REPETITIONS"

The claim: It's the optimal repetition range for building muscle.

The origin: In 1954, Ian MacQueen, MD, an English surgeon and competitive bodybuilder, published a scientific paper in which he recommended a moderately high number of repetitions for muscle growth.

The truth: This approach places the muscles under a medium amount of tension for a medium amount of time, making it both effective for and detrimental to maximum muscle gains.

A quick science lesson: Greater tension—a.k.a. heavier weights—induces the type of muscle growth in which the muscle fibers grow larger, leading to the best gains in strength; longer tension time, on the other hand, boosts muscle size by increasing the energy-producing structures around the fibers, improving muscular endurance. The classic prescription of 8 to 12 repetitions strikes a balance between the two. But by using that scheme all the time, you miss out on the greater tension levels that come with heavier weights and fewer repetitions, and the longer tension time achieved with lighter weights and more repetitions.

The new standard: Vary your repetition range—adjusting the weights accordingly—so that you stimulate every type of muscle growth. Try this method for a month, performing three full-body sessions a week: Do 5 repetitions per set in your first workout, 10 reps per set in your second workout, and 15 per set in your third workout.

THE AGE-OLD ADVICE: "DO THREE SETS OF EACH EXERCISE"

The claim: This provides the ideal workload for achieving the fastest muscle gains.

The origin: In 1948, a physician named Thomas Delorme reported in the *Archives of Physical Medicine* that performing three sets of 10 repetitions was as effective at improving leg strength as 10 sets of 10 repetitions.

The truth: There's nothing wrong with—or magical about—doing three sets. But the number of sets you perform shouldn't be determined by a 50-year-old default recommendation. Here's a rule of thumb: The more repetitions of an exercise you do, the fewer sets you should perform, and vice versa. This keeps the total number of reps you do of an exercise nearly equal, no matter how many repetitions make up each set.

The new standard: Use this chart to determine the number of sets you should do.

REPS	13–20	8–12	4–7	1–3
SETS	1–2	2–3	4–5	6–10

THE AGE-OLD ADVICE: "YOU NEED TO DO THREE OR FOUR EXERCISES PER MUSCLE GROUP"

The claim: This ensures that you work all the fibers of the target muscle.

The origin: Arnold, circa 1966.

The truth: You'll waste a lot of time. Here's why: Schwarzenegger's 4-decade-old recommendation is almost always combined with "Do three sets of 8 to 12 repetitions." That means you'll complete up to 144 repetitions for each muscle group. Trouble is, if you can perform even close to 100 repetitions for any muscle group, you're not working hard enough. Think of it this way: The harder you train, the less time you'll be able to sustain that level of effort. For example, many men can run for an hour if they jog slowly, but you'd be hard-pressed to find anyone who could do high-intensity sprints—without a major decrease in performance—for that period of time. And once performance starts to decline, you've achieved all the muscle-building benefits you can for that muscle group.

The new standard: Instead of focusing on the number of different exercises you do, shoot for a total number of repetitions between 25 and 50. That could mean five sets of five repetitions of one exercise (25 repetitions) or one set of 15 repetitions of two or three exercises (30 to 45 repetitions).

THE AGE-OLD ADVICE: "NEVER LET YOUR KNEES GO PAST YOUR TOES"

The claim: Allowing your knees to move too far forward during exercises such as the squat and lunge places dangerous shearing forces on your knee ligaments.

The origin: A 1978 study at Duke University found that keeping the lower leg as vertical as possible during the squat reduced shearing forces on the knee.

The truth: Leaning forward too much is more likely to cause injury. In 2003, University of Memphis researchers confirmed that knee stress was 28 percent higher when the knees were allowed to move past the toes during the squat. But the researchers also found a counter effect: Hip stress increased nearly 1,000 percent when forward movement of the knee was restricted. The reason: The squatters had to lean their torsos farther forward. And that's a problem, because forces that act on the hip are transferred to the lower back, a more frequent site of injury than the knees.

The new standard: Focus more on your upper body and less on knee position. By trying to keep your torso as upright as possible as you perform squats (and lunges), you'll reduce the stress on your hips and back. Two tips for staying upright: Before squatting, squeeze your shoulder blades together and hold them that way; and as you squat, try to keep your forearms perpendicular to the floor.

THE AGE-OLD ADVICE: "WHEN YOU LIFT WEIGHTS, DRAW IN YOUR ABS"

The claim: You'll increase the support to your spine, reducing the risk of back injuries.

The origin: In 1999, researchers in Australia found that some men with back pain had a slight delay in activating their transverse abdominis, a deep abdominal muscle that's part of the musculature that maintains spine stability. As a result, many fitness professionals began instructing their clients to try to pull their belly buttons to their spines—which engages the transverse abdominis—as they performed exercises.

The truth: "The research was accurate, but the interpretation by many researchers and therapists wasn't," says Stuart McGill, PhD, author of *Ultimate Back Fitness and Performance* and widely recognized as the world's top researcher on the spine. That's because muscles work in teams to stabilize your spine, and the most valuable players change depending on the exercise, says Dr. McGill. Read: The transverse abdominis isn't always the quarterback. In fact, for any given exercise, your body automatically activates the muscles that are most needed for spine support. So focusing only on your transverse abdominis can overrecruit the wrong muscles and underrecruit the right ones. This not only increases injury risk, but reduces the amount of weight you can lift.

The new standard: If you want to give your back a supporting hand, simply "brace" your abs as if you were about to be punched in the gut, but don't draw them in. "This activates all three layers of the abdominal wall, improving both stability and performance," says Dr. McGill.

PERFECT FORM

Iron out lifting flaws to get the most from these major muscle makers.

Barbell Squat

DON'T lean forward and bend down a few inches. This puts excessive pressure on your lower back while increasing the stress on your knees.

DO sit back (keep your torso as upright as possible) as you lower your body until your thighs are at least parallel to the floor.

Barbell Bench Press

DON'T overarch your back or lift your heels off the floor.

DO keep your back naturally arched (the way it is when you first lie down on the bench) and your feet flat on the floor at all times.

Dumbbell Shoulder Press

DON'T clank the weights together at the top of the movement; it increases risk of a shoulder-impingement injury without benefiting your muscles.

DO push the weights straight above your shoulders.

Chinup

DON'T stop partway down or use momentum to pull yourself back up.

DO lower your body until your arms are straight, pause, and then pull yourself back up.

SIMPLE SOLUTIONS FOR OUR FAVORITE EXCUSES

First, the legitimate excuses for skipping your workout. We found four: You're sore, you're sick, you're exhausted, you're hurt. That's it.

Soreness means your body needs a break: "Recovery is as important as working out," says Carter Hays, CSCS, a Houston-based personal trainer. Overtraining keeps as many men from reaching their goals as undertraining does, says Hays. An illness means you should knock off and let your body fight the bug. If you're so tired you're drowsy, you could hurt yourself. And if you're injured—especially if you're experiencing joint pain—let your body heal.

As for the rest of the excuses, listen up:

"Looks like rain." *Men's Health* cover model Gregg Avedon lives in Florida. Do the names Charley, Frances, Ivan, and Jeanne mean anything to you? Avedon spent much of 2004 lifting storm shutters and storing away patio furniture, then taking cover. He still looks great. Avedon says your home gym—those dumbbells over there, and

your chinup bar—makes staying inside a viable option. You can also spice up your indoor cardio by jumping rope or running up and down stairs. Or tie both ends of a resistance band to a doorway, place a towel across your chest, face away from the door with the band (cushioned by the towel) across your chest, and run in place.

"I have no time." Combine things you do anyway—work, breathe—with athletics. Set up business meetings during which you walk or jog; play tennis with your date; take a spin class to find dates; or take your family hiking, suggests Charles Stuart Platkin, MPH, author of *The Automatic Diet.*

"I pack my gym bag and then *Heroes* comes on." Get TiVo. Then tell yourself you're going to do just half of your regular routine. "It won't seem so insurmountable, and you'll end up doing the whole workout," says Edward Abramson, PhD, a clinical psychologist in Lafayette, California.

"I need my sleep." Pat Croce manages to stick with his workouts, and this father of two has been busy hosting his syndicated TV show, *Pat Croce: Moving In*, and opening a pirate museum in Key West, Florida. "Like me, you have to schedule fitness," he says. On the first of each month, Croce reviews his schedule with his secretary and then his wife, and breaks it down into weeks. Every Sunday, he goes over the coming week, making sure there are gyms at hotels where he'll be staying.

"I don't want to spend $50 a month on a gym membership." Don't. January's the month to negotiate fees, trial months, or group discounts. Think you don't have the cash? Save $900 a year by switching from a grande Guatemala Antigua to metabolism-boosting green tea when you stop at Starbucks every morning.

"My gym sucks." So move. Changing gyms is an opportunity for you to upgrade your workout. See the next tip.

"I'm bored with my workout." "Throw it in reverse," says Gunnar Peterson, CSCS, author of *G-Force*. If you always do lat pulldowns with an overhand grip, switch to underhand. Do a reverse-grip bench press, reverse-grip curls, reverse-grip triceps push-downs. Do front squats, rear lunges, and dumbbell lateral raises with your palms up. Count backward, too. "It's like a blastoff," says Peterson: "5, 4, 3, 2, 1, done."

"I never see results." Maybe you're not looking in the right places. Measure your waist, your heart rate, and your weight. Write them down. Then measure again after a week or two, says Croce. Celebrate even the smallest sign of progress. Muscles appear as fat melts.

"Four weeks, and no change in waistline, heart rate, or weight!" Whether you see results or not, you're strengthening your joints and connective tissues, which means you're laying down a foun-

dation for future muscle growth, says Peterson. Your diet, stress, sleep patterns, and other factors besides your workout may be holding you back—so don't give up.

"I have no energy." Eat. You need the fuel. "An active guy needs up to 1,000 calories more than an inactive guy," says Gay Riley, RD.

"I'm just making sure my body is getting adequate time to recover." After 72 hours of rest, you're just sliding backward. "But are you actually giving yourself a chance to recover?" asks Peterson. It's not all about time. Mix L-glutamine into your postworkout shake and eat a diet full of omega-3 fatty acids; they can assist with cellular reconstruction and the removal of metabolic wastes to help you recover faster, Peterson says.

"I always get hurt." This happens when you ratchet up your workout. Focus on losing 1 pound at a time or boosting your weights in 5-pound increments, says C.J. Murphy, MFS, owner of Total Performance Sports in Everett, Massachusetts. If you're used to doing 20 minutes on the treadmill, don't try a 2-hour road run. If you bench-press 50-pound dumbbells, don't go for 90. Instead, make small increases in the difficulty of your workout, focus on form, and work with a spotter so you still have a safety net, Murphy says.

"My elbows/shins/pinkie toes hurt." "Pain is a sure sign something is awry with your exercise choices," says Murphy. This year, don't isolate body parts so much—your muscles should function as a team. If your shoulder hurts for a week after you do lateral raises, stop doing them. Find a variation that doesn't cause pain, he says.

"I don't want to look stupid trying to use those space-age machines." Approach new machines with enthusiasm. "That's a good way to broaden your fitness spectrum," says Peterson. Read the placard, ask a trainer for assistance, and give it a shot. Nobody's looking. "They're so into themselves that they're not even thinking about you," Peterson says.

"I'm bored again." Organize your workout differently for 1 to 2 weeks, says Peterson. Let's say you're usually a push-pull guy—you do chinups and leg curls one workout, bench presses and squats another. Try working antagonistic, or opposing, muscle groups, such as your back and chest. You can also change to an upper/lower split routine in which you alternate upper-body workouts with lower-body ones. Or try a total-body workout a few times a week.

"My buddy can't make it tonight." It's easy to blame others. "If you're serious about training, think of it like a job," says Murphy. "If your training partner was an employee who continually was late and had poor performance, what would you do? You'd fire him!"

"I hate working out alone." Go to the gym at the same time and on the same days. Say hi to people. You'll find others who are on your schedule, says Dr. Abramson.

"I should really stay with my wife tonight and help with the baby. Plus, _Heroes_ is on." Or you could help all three of you. More and more gyms have childcare centers so you and your wife can get away and spend time together—something that new parents need, says Dr. Abramson. Or go over the calendar with your wife: For every day she's out, you can schedule a workout.

"Everyone's going out for drinks." Join them once a week "and you won't appear standoffish," Dr. Abramson says. But eat first. By having your drinks with a meal, you won't drink, snack, and eat dinner later.

"But _Heroes_ is on!" "Create a commitment you can't get out of," says Platkin. Make an appointment with a trainer who will charge you whether you show or not.

"I commute for an hour. I'm not getting back in my car." Go straight from work twice a week, then work out at home the other nights.

LOG WEEKS 1 TO 52

| WEEK 1 | WEEK OF / / TO / / | DAY: |

STRENGTH TRAINING

EXERCISE	WEIGHT	WARMUP SETS			WORK SETS		
		SET 1 REPS	SET 2 REPS	SET 3 REPS	SET 1 REPS	SET 2 REPS	SET 3 REPS

NOTES:

CARDIO

TYPE	INTENSITY	DURATION

NOTES:

THE AVERAGE GUY: HOW'S HE SHAPING UP?

Age when the average guy is in the best shape of his life: 23

Percentage of men who consider themselves "physically fit": 69

Percentage who actually are: 13

Time it takes the average guy to run a mile: 8 minutes, 34 seconds

Amount he can bench-press: 135 pounds

Number of situps he can do: 36

Pushups: 27

Pullups: 1

Size of the average guy's biceps: 11 inches

Size of his chest: 40 inches

Size of his waist: 34 inches

Percentage of men who don't belong to a gym: 88

Resting heart rate of a fit man: 52 beats per minute (bpm)

Resting heart rate of a man who's out of shape: 72 bpm

ARE YOU LIFTING ENOUGH WEIGHT?

Many men—beginners especially—might not be lifting as much as necessary to build muscle. Researchers at Grand Valley State University in Allendale, Michigan, asked 30 novices to work out with amounts of weight that they thought would help their muscles grow. All of the men chose weight loads below 60 percent of their one-repetition maximums (the heaviest you can lift once). "Lifting less than 60 percent will cause little tissue adaptation," says Stephen Glass, PhD, the lead study author. If you work with only 60 percent of your one-rep max using proper form, he says, you'll probably be able to do 15 to 20 repetitions. To build muscle, you should use weights that won't allow you to do that many.

WEEK 1 WEEK OF / / TO / /   DAY:

STRENGTH TRAINING

EXERCISE	WEIGHT	WARMUP SETS			WORK SETS		
		SET 1 REPS	SET 2 REPS	SET 3 REPS	SET 1 REPS	SET 2 REPS	SET 3 REPS

NOTES:

CARDIO

TYPE	INTENSITY	DURATION

NOTES:

SPOTLIGHT EXERCISE

TRIPLE-STOP PUSHUP

Assume the starting position of a regular pushup. Bend your arms to lower yourself halfway, then pause for 2 seconds.

Continue until your chest is just off the floor and hold again for 2 seconds. As you push yourself up, pause again for 2 seconds at the halfway point. Finally, when you straighten your arms, hold them that way—with your elbows unlocked—for 2 seconds. That's one repetition.

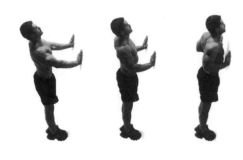

WEEK 1 | WEEK OF / / TO / / | DAY:

STRENGTH TRAINING

EXERCISE	WEIGHT	WARMUP SETS			WORK SETS		
		SET 1 REPS	SET 2 REPS	SET 3 REPS	SET 1 REPS	SET 2 REPS	SET 3 REPS

NOTES: _____

CARDIO

TYPE	INTENSITY	DURATION

NOTES: _____

BURN MORE FAT IN THE GYM

Where you sit when you work out could determine how fast you lose your gut. Irish researchers recently reported that men burn more fat while rowing than while biking. In the study, scientists measured the amount of fat used for fuel while men exercised on either a rowing machine or a stationary bike. The result: Participants burned 40 to 50 percent more fat when rowing than when cycling, even though the duration of exercise was the same. The likely explanation is that because rowing machines incorporate both your upper and lower body, they work more muscle, says lead study investigator David Ashley.

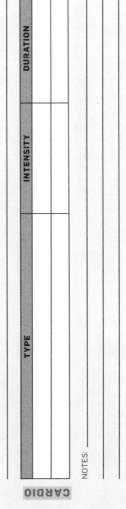

| WEEK 1 | WEEK OF / / TO / / | DAY: |

STRENGTH TRAINING

EXERCISE	WEIGHT	WARMUP SETS			WORK SETS		
		SET 1 REPS	SET 2 REPS	SET 3 REPS	SET 1 REPS	SET 2 REPS	SET 3 REPS

NOTES: _____

CARDIO

TYPE	INTENSITY	DURATION

NOTES: _____

SCULPT AND STRENGTHEN

DEVELOP A FASTER FIRST STEP

Quickness like Dwyane Wade's requires exercises that force you to push off the inside and outside of your foot. Try the staggered-stance forward long jump and lateral long jump. With your legs slightly bent and feet hip-width apart, project your hips forward for the forward jump and laterally for the lateral jump. For the forward jump, stagger your feet. A split stance trains your nervous system to recruit muscle fibers as if you were running, says Jon Crosby, CSCS, who works with NFL players. Alternate which foot is forward. Do four sets of five repetitions of each exercise, resting for 20 seconds between jumps and 60 seconds between sets.

WEEK 2 | WEEK OF / / TO / / | DAY:

STRENGTH TRAINING

EXERCISE	WEIGHT	WARMUP SETS			WORK SETS		
		SET 1 REPS	SET 2 REPS	SET 3 REPS	SET 1 REPS	SET 2 REPS	SET 3 REPS

NOTES: _____

CARDIO

TYPE	INTENSITY	DURATION

NOTES: _____

TRAINING TIP
DOUBLE YOUR GAINS

Your high-school football coach was onto something with two-a-days. New research finds that splitting your cardio workout into two sessions could double your fitness gains. University of New Hampshire researchers divided 37 people into two groups and had them do aerobic workouts 4 days a week. One group exercised once a day for 30 minutes, while the other exercised twice a day for 15 minutes at a time. After 12 weeks, the twice-a-day exercisers had increased their workout capacity by 21 percent and VO₂ max by 9 percent—double the results of the once-a-day group. Author Timothy Quinn, PhD, says the twice-a-day group stayed warmed up between sessions and were able to attack the second workout. Also, the shorter workout duration meant they didn't tire and could spend more time in a higher heart-rate zone.

WEEK 2 | WEEK OF / / TO / / | DAY:

STRENGTH TRAINING

EXERCISE	WEIGHT	WARMUP SETS			WORK SETS		
		SET 1 REPS	SET 2 REPS	SET 3 REPS	SET 1 REPS	SET 2 REPS	SET 3 REPS

NOTES:

CARDIO

TYPE	INTENSITY	DURATION

NOTES:

CHINUP CHALLENGE

Unlock the Best Back Exercise

CHINUP

Do as many chinups as you can. Rest, then do another set of one less than your max. Perform a third set of two less than your max.

DUMBBELL ROW

Grab two heavy dumbbells with an underhand grip, knees slightly bent. With your torso almost parallel to the floor, pull one weight up until your elbow is higher than your torso, then lower it. Do three sets of six reps per arm.

BICEPS CURL

Hold dumbbells at arm's length, palms forward. Keeping your upper arms against your sides, curl the weights toward your shoulders. Squeeze your biceps, then lower the weights. Do three sets of six reps.

WEEK 2   WEEK OF / / TO / /   DAY: ____

STRENGTH TRAINING

EXERCISE	WEIGHT	WARMUP SETS			WORK SETS		
		SET 1 REPS	SET 2 REPS	SET 3 REPS	SET 1 REPS	SET 2 REPS	SET 3 REPS

NOTES: _____

CARDIO

TYPE	INTENSITY	DURATION

NOTES: _____

FUELING UP

UPGRADE YOUR BREAKFAST

You need at least 30 grams of protein per meal for your body to maximize the muscle-building process, suggest researchers at the University of Illinois at Urbana-Champaign. These simple recipes pack extra protein.

Power Oatmeal

- ½ cup oat bran
- ½ cup oats
- ⅓ cup water
- 1 scoop chocolate whey-protein powder

Nuke the oat bran, oats, and water for 3 to 4 minutes. Stir in the protein powder.

Speed Shake

- 1 scoop vanilla whey-protein powder
- ½ cup oats
- Milk or water

Add protein powder and oats to a shaker bottle. Pour in milk or water, shake, and drink.

Muscle Toast

- 6 ounces Atlantic salmon (try Bumble Bee wild salmon)
- 1 slice whole wheat toast

Place the salmon on the toast and eat.

WEEK 2 | **WEEK OF** / / **TO** / / | **DAY:**

STRENGTH TRAINING

EXERCISE	WEIGHT	WARMUP SETS			WORK SETS		
		SET 1 REPS	SET 2 REPS	SET 3 REPS	SET 1 REPS	SET 2 REPS	SET 3 REPS

NOTES: _____

CARDIO

TYPE	INTENSITY	DURATION

NOTES: _____

COUNT DOWN TO BULK UP

You know building muscle takes time. But how long? About 3 weeks, according to U.K. researchers. In a recent study, the scientists determined that visible muscle growth occurs after just 20 days of heavy weight training. In fact, the researchers found that by doing four sets of seven reps of leg extensions 3 days a week, the lifters increased quadriceps muscle size by about 0.2 percent a day. Even though this growth isn't noticeable from day to day, the effect can be dramatic if you work all your major muscle groups 3 days a week, 52 weeks a year. In the past year, have you trained your entire body 156 times?

WEEK 3 | WEEK OF / / TO / / | DAY:

STRENGTH TRAINING

EXERCISE	WEIGHT	WARMUP SETS			WORK SETS		
		SET 1 REPS	SET 2 REPS	SET 3 REPS	SET 1 REPS	SET 2 REPS	SET 3 REPS

NOTES:

CARDIO

TYPE	INTENSITY	DURATION

NOTES:

TRAINING TIP
START EXPLOSIVELY

Don't always lead with your hardest exercise. Try an explosive movement before a traditional strength exercise. In a study published in the *Journal of Strength and Conditioning Research*, men who did a squat after a hang clean—an explosive move used by Olympic lifters—performed better than men who squatted to start their workouts. Why? They were able to generate more power. The researchers speculate that performing an explosive exercise first causes chemical changes to occur at the level of the muscle fiber, stimulating a greater number of nerves to activate during the second movement. See for yourself: Before a set of squats, do jump squats—bend at the hips and knees to lower your body about 6 inches, then push off forcefully so your feet leave the floor.

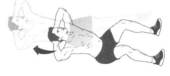

WEEK 3	WEEK OF / / TO / /	DAY:

STRENGTH TRAINING

EXERCISE	WEIGHT	WARMUP SETS			WORK SETS		
		SET 1 REPS	SET 2 REPS	SET 3 REPS	SET 1 REPS	SET 2 REPS	SET 3 REPS

NOTES:

CARDIO

TYPE	INTENSITY	DURATION

NOTES:

Ask the Trainer

If you had time to do only three exercises, what would they be?

—Martin, Columbia, SC

You can't go wrong with bench presses, deadlifts, and pullups—they work so much mass and ignite a surge of muscle-building hormones. But my three must-have moves include none of them. One essential is the squat-and-press. It does wonders for fat loss, because you work your upper and lower body in one motion. Another big hitter is the Swiss-ball pushup. Say what you want about Swiss balls, this spin on a classic exercise adds some much-needed core action to a proven chest-and-shoulder builder. Finally, make sure you have the inverted row in your arsenal. It strengthens the muscles that pull your shoulder blades back into their proper position, so it helps correct and perfect your posture.

WEEK 3 | WEEK OF / / TO / / | DAY:

STRENGTH TRAINING

| EXERCISE | WEIGHT | WARM-UP SETS | | | WORK SETS | | |
		SET 1 REPS	SET 2 REPS	SET 3 REPS	SET 1 REPS	SET 2 REPS	SET 3 REPS

NOTES:

CARDIO

TYPE	INTENSITY	DURATION

NOTES:

CORE POWER

YOUR MUSCLES IN MOTION

RECTUS ABDOMINIS

You might want a six-pack, but the rectus abdominis is actually made up of four sections and a tendon called the linea alba that divides them into two parts—creating an eight-pack.

OBLIQUES

Forget the fallacy that building your obliques will give you a wider-looking waist. Strong obliques help you rotate your torso with more force, allowing you to be more active and burn more calories in any sport.

HIP FLEXORS

For many men, the psoas—a core muscle that attaches to your upper thigh—is both tight and weak, which is why moves like the lunge lift are essential. They stretch and strengthen your hip flexors.

WEEK 3   WEEK OF / / TO / /   DAY:

STRENGTH TRAINING

EXERCISE	WEIGHT	WARMUP SETS			WORK SETS		
		SET 1 REPS	SET 2 REPS	SET 3 REPS	SET 1 REPS	SET 2 REPS	SET 3 REPS

NOTES:

CARDIO

TYPE	INTENSITY	DURATION

NOTES:

WEEK 4 | WEEK OF / / TO / / | DAY:

STRENGTH TRAINING

EXERCISE	WEIGHT	WARMUP SETS			WORK SETS		
		SET 1 REPS	SET 2 REPS	SET 3 REPS	SET 1 REPS	SET 2 REPS	SET 3 REPS

NOTES: _____

CARDIO

TYPE	INTENSITY	DURATION

NOTES: _____

FUELING UP

WHOLE GRAINS FOR BIGGER WEIGHT-LOSS GAINS

It's not a magic disappearing act, but it's close. Adding a bowl of oatmeal to your daily diet can help keep off the pounds. When Harvard University researchers analyzed the diets of more than 27,000 men over 8 years, they discovered that the men who added one serving of whole grain foods daily weighed 2.5 pounds less than the men who ate only refined-grain foods. The high fiber helped, but the benefits went beyond simple satiety. "Whole grains may more favorably affect blood-glucose levels," says Pauline Koh-Banerjee, ScD, the study author. If you miss your whole grains at breakfast, try again at dinner; 90 seconds is all you'll need to nuke a three-quarter-cup serving of Uncle Ben's new heat-and-eat brown rice.

Ask the Trainer

Girls like a nice butt. I want girls. Help me out.
—Lee, Simi Valley, CA

Try this sequence from Carter Hays, CSCS.

Hold a pair of light dumbbells at your sides. Standing straight, step forward with your left foot until your back knee is an inch off the floor and your front knee is over (not past) your toes. Push back to the starting position, then press the weights overhead. Repeat with your right foot. Next, lunge out to your left, then return to the starting position and press the weights overhead. Repeat on your right. Repeat with each leg lunging straight back, following with a shoulder press. Perform this sequence three times before your leg workouts for 6 weeks.

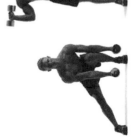

| WEEK 4 | WEEK OF / / TO / / | DAY: |

STRENGTH TRAINING

EXERCISE	WEIGHT	WARMUP SETS			WORK SETS		
		SET 1 REPS	SET 2 REPS	SET 3 REPS	SET 1 REPS	SET 2 REPS	SET 3 REPS

NOTES: _____

CARDIO

TYPE	INTENSITY	DURATION

NOTES: _____

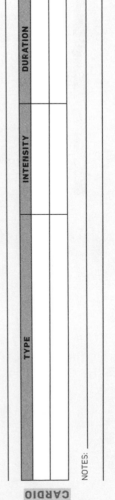

FITNESS FACT

GOOD THINGS COME TO THOSE WHO WAIT

Just wait—your bench press will improve. University of Kansas researchers studied 28 men performing sets of bench presses to failure. The men who rested for at least 3 minutes between sets performed 32 percent better in the second set than those who rested for only a minute. "When muscle fatigues, the concentration of hydrogen ions in the muscle rises, which can make it harder to produce force," says Michael Godard, PhD, the senior study author and director of the university's applied-physiology laboratory. This concentration decreases with rest. The researchers also found that resting for 5 minutes between sets did not improve performance any more than the 3-minute break did.

WEEK 4	WEEK OF / / TO / /	DAY:

STRENGTH TRAINING

EXERCISE	WEIGHT	WARMUP SETS			WORK SETS		
		SET 1 REPS	SET 2 REPS	SET 3 REPS	SET 1 REPS	SET 2 REPS	SET 3 REPS

NOTES: _____

CARDIO

TYPE	INTENSITY	DURATION

NOTES: _____

TRAINING TIP
BUILD BIGGER ARMS

Speed up. When researchers at the University of Sydney had two groups of men perform biceps curls at either a slow tempo (3 seconds up, 3 seconds down) or a fast tempo (1 second up, 1 second down), they found that lifting fast builds 11 percent more strength than training at slow speeds. "Changing the speed of reps either from workout to workout or from set to set can build muscle," says Matthew Rhea, PhD. Try it: For the next 4 weeks, add a set of six to eight biceps curls to your workout 3 days a week. Use the heaviest weight that allows you to complete the reps fast without having to lean forward or back.

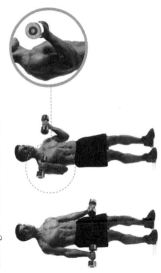

WEEK 4 | **WEEK OF** / / **TO** / / | **DAY:**

STRENGTH TRAINING

EXERCISE	WEIGHT	WARMUP SETS						WORK SETS					
		SET 1		SET 2		SET 3		SET 1		SET 2		SET 3	
		REPS		REPS		REPS		REPS		REPS		REPS	

NOTES: _____

CARDIO

TYPE	INTENSITY	DURATION

NOTES: _____

SCULPT AND STRENGTHEN

Perform better with this hybrid exercise (two or more movements that merge). Do three sets of 8 to 10 repetitions of each hybrid exercise below, resting 1 to 2 minutes between sets:

ROTATIONAL REACH-AND-TOUCH LUNGE TO CURL AND PRESS

Stand holding dumbbells at your sides. With your left leg, lunge forward and to the left at a 45-degree angle. (1) As you bend your knee to lower your body, reach with both arms and touch the weights to the floor, one on each side of your left foot. (2) As you push yourself up, curl the weights to your shoulders, (3) then press them overhead. (4) Return to the starting position. That's one rep. Repeat for a total of 8 to 10, alternating legs as you go.

WEEK 5 | WEEK OF / / TO / / | DAY:

STRENGTH TRAINING

EXERCISE	WEIGHT	WARMUP SETS						WORK SETS					
		SET 1		SET 2		SET 3		SET 1		SET 2		SET 3	
		REPS		REPS		REPS		REPS		REPS		REPS	

NOTES: _____

CARDIO

TYPE	INTENSITY	DURATION

NOTES: _____

CORE POWER

SQUAT FOR A SIX-PACK

If you're not doing squats for your legs, consider using them to sculpt your midsection. When Canadian researchers measured abdominal-muscle activity during several popular exercises, they determined that squats work your core harder than many ab and lower-back exercises. Although squatting with the heaviest weights stimulated the most muscle, even lightweight warmup sets targeted the men's abs intensely.

WEEK 5 | **WEEK OF** / / **TO** / / | **DAY:**

STRENGTH TRAINING

EXERCISE	WEIGHT	WARMUP SETS			WORK SETS		
		SET 1 REPS	SET 2 REPS	SET 3 REPS	SET 1 REPS	SET 2 REPS	SET 3 REPS

NOTES:

CARDIO

TYPE	INTENSITY	DURATION

NOTES:

TRAINING TIP

SET A NEW BENCHMARK

How much did your bench press increase last year? Don't settle for satisfactory progress, even if you think your strength has peaked. In a recent study, Australian researchers found that even experienced lifters can boost their bench presses by 64 pounds in 4 years. Consider this a long-term goal for yourself. Break it down to a manageable 16 pounds a year and start chipping away with our strength-building workouts.

WEEK 5 | WEEK OF / / TO / / | DAY:

STRENGTH TRAINING

EXERCISE	WEIGHT	WARMUP SETS			WORK SETS		
		SET 1 REPS	SET 2 REPS	SET 3 REPS	SET 1 REPS	SET 2 REPS	SET 3 REPS

NOTES:

CARDIO

TYPE	INTENSITY	DURATION

NOTES:

SPOTLIGHT EXERCISE

STANDING HAMMER CURL

Place this exercise at the end of your arm workout, so your forearms aren't fatigued for other exercises. Two common mistakes are swinging your body so momentum cheats the weight up, and allowing gravity to lower the weight too quickly. Leaning backward and forward not only stresses your lower back, but also cheats your arms. Use weights that allow you to maintain perfect form.

1. Stand with your feet slightly less than shoulder-width apart and hold a pair of dumbbells at your sides with a neutral grip (palms facing you).

2. Keeping your abs drawn in, your back straight, and your elbows at your sides, raise your forearms. Don't let your shoulders or elbows move forward, and watch that your elbows don't move outward.

3. When the dumbbells are just in front of your shoulders, take 2 to 3 seconds to lower the weights until your arms are straight. Come to a full stop at the bottom of the movement before repeating.

WEEK 5   WEEK OF / / TO / /   DAY:

STRENGTH TRAINING

EXERCISE	WEIGHT	WARMUP SETS			WORK SETS		
		SET 1 REPS	SET 2 REPS	SET 3 REPS	SET 1 REPS	SET 2 REPS	SET 3 REPS

NOTES:

CARDIO

TYPE	INTENSITY	DURATION

NOTES:

SCULPT AND STRENGTHEN

BUILD A BEACH-READY BODY

Rest for 15 seconds after each exercise and 60 seconds after the circuit. Repeat twice.

JUMPING ROPE

Jump rope for 90 seconds. Hop on one leg, alternating between legs. Jump once on your right foot, once on your left, twice on your right, twice on your left, etc., until you're alternating every 10 jumps between right and left.

SHUTTLE RUN

Position five small objects in a row 10 to 15 yards away from you. Sprint toward the objects and bring them back to the starting line one by one as quickly as possible.

SQUAT THRUST

From a standing position, bend at the hips and knees to lower yourself into a deep squat. Place your hands on the floor in front of you, then kick your legs back so you're in pushup position. Immediately bring your legs forward again so you're back in squat position and stand up. Perform 10 squats.

FOOTBALL RUNDOWN

On a large field, throw or kick a football as far as you can. Run to retrieve it, then repeat. Do six to eight reps.

WEEK 6 WEEK OF / / TO / / DAY:

STRENGTH TRAINING

EXERCISE	WEIGHT	WARMUP SETS						WORK SETS					
		SET 1		SET 2		SET 3		SET 1		SET 2		SET 3	
		REPS		REPS		REPS		REPS		REPS		REPS	

NOTES:

CARDIO

TYPE	INTENSITY	DURATION

NOTES:

Ask the Trainer

How should I adjust my workout to get ready for warm-weather sports like softball and golf?
—*Y.T., Piscataway, NJ*

If you're ramping up for any activity that requires strenuous arm and shoulder work—throwing, swinging, even pulling ropes on a sailboat—you have to work your rotator cuffs. To do that, add to your workout the rotational pushup on a medicine ball.

Get into a pushup position with your right hand on the floor and your left hand on a medicine ball. (1) As you straighten your arms, lift your right hand off the floor and raise it until your right arm points toward the ceiling. (2) Keep your back straight and don't bend your knees—you want to make your left arm work harder to stabilize on the medicine ball. After a set of 8 to 10, switch arms and repeat.

WEEK 6 | WEEK OF / / TO / / | DAY:

STRENGTH TRAINING

EXERCISE	WEIGHT	WARMUP SETS			WORK SETS		
		SET 1 REPS	SET 2 REPS	SET 3 REPS	SET 1 REPS	SET 2 REPS	SET 3 REPS

NOTES:

CARDIO

TYPE	INTENSITY	DURATION

NOTES:

WEEK 6 | WEEK OF / / TO / / | DAY:

EXERCISE	WEIGHT	WARMUP SETS			WORK SETS		
		SET 1 REPS	SET 2 REPS	SET 3 REPS	SET 1 REPS	SET 2 REPS	SET 3 REPS

NOTES: _____

TYPE	INTENSITY	DURATION

NOTES: _____

STRETCH IT OUT

STRETCH FOR STRENGTH

Poor desk posture and too much bench-pressing cause "adaptive shortening" of the pectoral muscles, making it harder to build strength and size. The following low-cable moves restore range of motion; do both before your chest routine.

SIDE-LYING REVERSE FLY

1. Attach a handle to the low pulley and lie on your right side facing the stack. (Use the lightest weight that lets you feel your back muscles contract.)

2. Grab the handle with your left hand and move your left arm upward and back behind your torso, then return to the starting position. Do 10 reps, then lie on your left side and repeat with your right arm.

LYING CHOP

1. Lie on your back with your head 2 feet in front of the stack. Grab the handle with your left hand, palm up. Hold your shoulder blades together throughout the move.

2. Pull the handle down and across your body to your right hip, rotating your arm so your palm ends up facing your hip. Pause, then reverse the movement, and repeat for a set of 10. Repeat with your right arm.

SPOTLIGHT EXERCISE

DUMBBELL PUSHUP ROW

Get into pushup position with your arms straight and your hands resting on light dumbbells.

Squeeze your abs and glutes as you perform a pushup.

At the top, pull one dumbbell off the floor and toward you until your elbow is above your back. Slowly return the weight to the floor and repeat with the other arm.

WEEK 6	WEEK OF / / TO / /	DAY:

STRENGTH TRAINING

EXERCISE	WEIGHT	WARMUP SETS			WORK SETS		
		SET 1 REPS	SET 2 REPS	SET 3 REPS	SET 1 REPS	SET 2 REPS	SET 3 REPS

NOTES:

CARDIO

TYPE	INTENSITY	DURATION

NOTES:

SCULPT AND STRENGTHEN

BUILD BIGGER BICEPS

ZOTTMAN CURL

1. Using dumbbells that are 5 to 10 pounds lighter than you normally use, lie faceup on a 45-degree incline bench. Hold the weights at your sides with an underhand grip (palms facing forward).

2. Curl the weights toward your shoulders.

3. Rotate your wrists at the top of the movement so your palms are facedown.

4. Lower the weights and turn your wrists at the bottom of the move to return to an underhand grip. Continue rotating and curling for three or four sets of six to eight reps.

1.

2.

3.

4.

WEEK 7 | WEEK OF / / TO / / | DAY:

STRENGTH TRAINING

EXERCISE	WEIGHT	WARMUP SETS						WORK SETS					
		SET 1		SET 2		SET 3		SET 1		SET 2		SET 3	
		REPS		REPS		REPS		REPS		REPS		REPS	

NOTES: _____
_____

CARDIO

TYPE	INTENSITY	DURATION

NOTES: _____
_____

SPOTLIGHT EXERCISE

OBLIQUE HANGING LEG RAISE

Grab a chinup bar with an overhand grip and hang from it at arm's length, with your knees bent and pulled up toward your chest. Keeping your knees bent and heels together, lift your left hip toward your left armpit until your lower legs are nearly parallel to the floor. Pause, then slowly return to the starting position. Then lift your right hip toward your right armpit. Continue to alternate until you've done 10 on each side. Perform three sets.

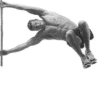

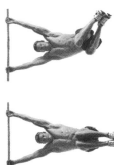

STRENGTH TRAINING

EXERCISE	WEIGHT	WARMUP SETS			WORK SETS		
		SET 1 REPS	SET 2 REPS	SET 3 REPS	SET 1 REPS	SET 2 REPS	SET 3 REPS

NOTES:

CARDIO

TYPE	INTENSITY	DURATION

NOTES:

BIG MUSCLES ON A BUDGET

Here's how to bulk up, no matter what your bankroll.

If you have $100, buy . . .

A Stability Ball Plus ($23, www.performbetter.com). Made of burst-resistant vinyl, this Swiss ball comes in four sizes and can hold up to 600 pounds.

A pair of Pro Style dumbbells ($70, www.performbetter.com).

If you have ANOTHER $160, add . . .

The HF-4163 flat bench from Hoist Fitness (www.hoistfitness.com), which adjusts for flat, incline, and decline exercises—and collapses to fit under a bed ($160).

If you have ANOTHER $400, buy . . .

A pair of Nautilus SelecTech Dumbbells. Twist the end caps to transform each dumbbell from 5 to 52.5 pounds and weights in between ($400, www.nautilus.com).

If you have ANOTHER $1,210, add . . .

A power rack/cage from Tuff Stuff ($550, www.tuffstuff.net) and a 300-pound weight set with bar from Ivanko weights ($660, www.ivanko.com).

WEEK 7 WEEK OF / / TO / / DAY:

STRENGTH TRAINING

EXERCISE	WEIGHT	WARMUP SETS			WORK SETS		
		SET 1 REPS	SET 2 REPS	SET 3 REPS	SET 1 REPS	SET 2 REPS	SET 3 REPS

NOTES:

CARDIO

TYPE	INTENSITY	DURATION

NOTES:

TRAINING TIP

BIG ARMS IN NO TIME

Once you're in the gym, you don't have to stay long. A Finnish study found that men gain the same levels of strength and build equal amounts of muscle whether they rest 2 minutes or 5 minutes between sets. Lead study author Juha Ahtiainen, PhD, says this finding can benefit men who would like faster workouts, as well as men who feel they need more time to rest between sets. "For practical purposes, just rest long enough to be mentally and physically ready for your next set," says Dr. Ahtiainen.

WEEK 7	WEEK OF / / TO / /	DAY:

STRENGTH TRAINING

EXERCISE	WEIGHT	WARMUP SETS						WORK SETS					
		SET 1		SET 2		SET 3		SET 1		SET 2		SET 3	
		REPS		REPS		REPS		REPS		REPS		REPS	

NOTES: _____

CARDIO

TYPE	INTENSITY	DURATION

NOTES: _____

| WEEK 8 | WEEK OF / / TO / / | DAY: |

STRENGTH TRAINING

EXERCISE	WEIGHT	WARMUP SETS			WORK SETS		
		SET 1 REPS	SET 2 REPS	SET 3 REPS	SET 1 REPS	SET 2 REPS	SET 3 REPS

NOTES: _____

CARDIO

TYPE	INTENSITY	DURATION

NOTES: _____

FUELING UP

EAT LIKE A COVER MODEL

Your heavy lifting is over when you leave the gym, but your body is just getting started, working furiously to replenish glycogen stores. This is why you should always eat a hearty serving of carbohydrates and protein after a workout—so your body can start building new muscle tissue fast. The fruits in this recipe contain enzymes to help your body quickly break down nutrients so they can be delivered to your muscles.

Postworkout Fruit Salad

1 cup Friendship brand 1% low-fat cottage cheese, no salt added (packs a whopping 32 grams of protein)

1 cup diced pineapple

1 cup diced papaya

1 kiwifruit, peeled and sliced

½ mango, peeled and diced

1 banana, sliced

1 tablespoon clover honey

When you return from the gym, dish out the cottage cheese and a serving of your fruit mix, and top with the honey. Not sweet enough? Add a sweetener like Equal, Splenda, or stevia.

FITNESS FACT

THE HIP FACTOR

The best solutions aren't always the most obvious: Doing exercises and stretches for your hips alleviates knee pain, according to new research in the *American Journal of Sports Medicine*. In the study, 35 men and women with chronic knee pain performed daily stretches and strengthening exercises for their hips. After 6 weeks, more than half of the patients had eliminated knee pain when squatting, sitting, and climbing stairs. One of their signature moves was the stepup: Holding a pair of dumbbells at your sides, stand facing a step or bench. Place one foot on the step and push down through your heel to lift your other leg up to the step. Return to the starting position and finish a set of 12 to 15 repetitions with one leg before switching legs and repeating the exercise.

WEEK 8 **WEEK OF** / / **TO** / / **DAY:**

STRENGTH TRAINING

EXERCISE	WEIGHT	WARMUP SETS						WORK SETS					
		SET 1		SET 2		SET 3		SET 1		SET 2		SET 3	
		REPS		REPS		REPS		REPS		REPS		REPS	

NOTES: _____

CARDIO

TYPE	INTENSITY	DURATION

NOTES: _____

BODY MOVING

RUN FOR BIG BICEPS

Cardio training can help you recover faster from strength workouts. In a study published in the *Journal of Strength and Conditioning Research*, researchers found that men with greater aerobic fitness were able to recover faster after bouts of resistance exercise. According to the study, cardio trains your body to remove metabolic waste products and replenish oxygen stores more efficiently, which helps you recover from any type of exercise.

WEEK 8   WEEK OF / / TO / /   DAY:

STRENGTH TRAINING

EXERCISE	WEIGHT	WARMUP SETS			WORK SETS		
		SET 1 REPS	SET 2 REPS	SET 3 REPS	SET 1 REPS	SET 2 REPS	SET 3 REPS

NOTES: _____

CARDIO

TYPE	INTENSITY	DURATION

NOTES: _____

TRAINING TIP

LIFT FIRST, RUN SECOND

We've long touted the fat-loss benefits of weight training. But now Japanese scientists have discovered that lifting weights before you run helps you burn more flab while you pound the pavement. In fact, men who performed a weight-lifting routine and then hopped on a stationary bike burned twice as much fat as those who only pedaled. Resistance exercise stimulates the release of fat-burning hormones, which trigger your body to use more lard for energy.

WEEK 8 | **WEEK OF** / / **TO** / / | **DAY:**

STRENGTH TRAINING

EXERCISE	WEIGHT	WARMUP SETS			WORK SETS		
		SET 1 REPS	SET 2 REPS	SET 3 REPS	SET 1 REPS	SET 2 REPS	SET 3 REPS

NOTES: _____

CARDIO

TYPE	INTENSITY	DURATION

NOTES: _____

FITNESS FACT

HEAD SOUTH THIS WINTER

In a recent study published in the *Journal of Applied Physiology*, scientists found that running downhill helps a rat develop its all-important spinotrapezius—a muscle with a fiber composition similar to that of the human quadriceps. For us, running on any decline stresses the quadriceps and gluteals, says study author David Poole, PhD. Running downhill puts these muscles under "almost three times as much force as level or uphill running" and builds the quads, Dr. Poole says.

WEEK 9	WEEK OF / / TO / /	DAY:

STRENGTH TRAINING

EXERCISE	WEIGHT	WARMUP SETS			WORK SETS		
		SET 1 REPS	SET 2 REPS	SET 3 REPS	SET 1 REPS	SET 2 REPS	SET 3 REPS

NOTES:

CARDIO

TYPE	INTENSITY	DURATION

NOTES:

SPOTLIGHT EXERCISE

EXPLOSIVE CROSSOVER PUSHUP

Place your right hand on the floor and your left hand on the smooth side of a weight plate. Lower your body.

Explosively push up and to the left so your hands leave the floor. Land with your right hand on the plate and your left hand on the floor. Reverse the move.

WEEK 9 WEEK OF / / TO / / DAY:

STRENGTH TRAINING

EXERCISE	WEIGHT	WARMUP SETS			WORK SETS		
		SET 1 REPS	SET 2 REPS	SET 3 REPS	SET 1 REPS	SET 2 REPS	SET 3 REPS

NOTES:

CARDIO

TYPE	INTENSITY	DURATION

NOTES:

| WEEK 9 | WEEK OF / / TO / / | DAY: |

STRENGTH TRAINING

		WARMUP SETS			WORK SETS		
		SET 1	SET 2	SET 3	SET 1	SET 2	SET 3
EXERCISE	WEIGHT	REPS	REPS	REPS	REPS	REPS	REPS

NOTES:

CARDIO

TYPE	INTENSITY	DURATION

NOTES:

FUELING UP
DRINK OF THE DAY

Scientists at Baylor University found that men who drink a mixture of carbohydrates and a special blend of protein after lifting weights gain 8 percent more muscle in 10 weeks than guys who don't down a shake. The formula: 5 grams carbohydrates, 24 grams whey protein, and 16 grams casein protein. A protein blend of fast-digesting whey and slow-digesting casein provides a steady supply of raw materials to the muscle, says lead researcher Darryn Willoughby, PhD. Go to www.proteinfactory.com to create a made-to-order protein powder.

FITNESS FACT
FOREVER LEAN

Weight training may turn back the clock. Here's the theory: If you could offset the natural decline in testosterone levels, you might be able to build more muscle, burn fat faster, and lift your libido. And though scientists have long known that resistance exercise boosts testosterone in young men after a workout, a new study in the *Journal of Strength and Conditioning Research* shows that this is true for men of all ages—even into your seventies. The next step is to determine whether this temporary rise has a lasting effect on a man's health.

WEEK 9   WEEK OF / / TO / /   DAY: [ ]

STRENGTH TRAINING

EXERCISE	WEIGHT	WARMUP SETS			WORK SETS		
		SET 1 REPS	SET 2 REPS	SET 3 REPS	SET 1 REPS	SET 2 REPS	SET 3 REPS

NOTES: _____

CARDIO

TYPE	INTENSITY	DURATION

NOTES: _____

BODY MOVING

TRAIN LIKE THE CHAMP

Give your workout a jump start with this drill from Shaun Hamilton, head coach of USA Jump Rope.

JOG STEP

Begin with your right foot planted, your left foot slightly above the floor, and the rope behind you. Swing the rope over your head, jump, and land on your right foot. As the rope comes down, jump off your right foot—allowing the rope to pass under both feet—and land on your left foot, keeping your right foot suspended.

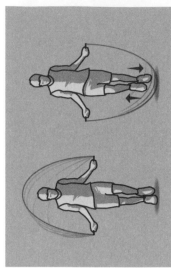

| WEEK 10 | WEEK OF / / TO / / | DAY: |

STRENGTH TRAINING

EXERCISE	WEIGHT	WARMUP SETS			WORK SETS		
		SET 1 REPS	SET 2 REPS	SET 3 REPS	SET 1 REPS	SET 2 REPS	SET 3 REPS

NOTES:

CARDIO

TYPE	INTENSITY	DURATION

NOTES:

WEEK 10 | WEEK OF / / TO / / | DAY:

STRENGTH TRAINING

EXERCISE	WEIGHT	WARMUP SETS			WORK SETS		
		SET 1 REPS	SET 2 REPS	SET 3 REPS	SET 1 REPS	SET 2 REPS	SET 3 REPS

NOTES:

CARDIO

TYPE	INTENSITY	DURATION

NOTES:

FUELING UP

THE WORST FOODS EVER

Three esteemed nutritionists tell the world which foods a man should never consume. Their opinions:

MARY ELLEN CAMIRE, PhD, professor of food science at the University of Maine in Orono:

Raw oysters. "They can be contaminated with hepatitis and other nasty viruses."

DAVID GROTTO, RD, director of nutrition education at the Block Center for Integrative Cancer Care in Evanston, Illinois:

Pork rinds. "They do give you protein, but so would eating your own skin."

DAVID KATZ, MD, director of medical studies in public health at Yale University and author of *The Way to Eat*:

Any processed lunch meat, such as corned beef, pastrami, or bologna. "These deli meats are loaded with saturated fat."

TRAINING TIP

BURN BLUBBER, NOT BICEPS

Weight training is a key ingredient in any belly-off plan. Case in point: Ball State University researchers put overweight men on a 1,500-calorie-a-day diet and divided them into three groups—one that didn't exercise, another that performed aerobic exercise 3 days a week, and a third that did aerobic exercise and weight training 3 days a week.

The results: Each group lost nearly the same amount of weight—about 21 pounds. But the lifters shed 5 pounds more fat than those who didn't pump iron. Why? Because their weight loss was almost pure fat, while the other two groups lost just 15 pounds of lard and several pounds of lean body mass, a.k.a. muscle.

Diet only: 69 percent fat mass

Diet + aerobic exercise: 78 percent fat mass

Diet + aerobic exercise + weight training: 97 percent fat mass

---

WEEK 10 **WEEK OF** / / **TO** / / **DAY:**

STRENGTH TRAINING

EXERCISE	WEIGHT	WARMUP SETS						WORK SETS					
		SET 1		SET 2		SET 3		SET 1		SET 2		SET 3	
		REPS		REPS		REPS		REPS		REPS		REPS	

NOTES: _____

CARDIO

TYPE	INTENSITY	DURATION

NOTES: _____

FUELING UP

MILK, FOR ALL IT'S WORTH

What do you reach for after a hard run? Not a carton of chocolate milk? Consider it next time. A new study concludes that chocolate milk is an effective postexercise drink that speeds recovery. According to the *International Journal of Sport Nutrition and Exercise Metabolism*, Indiana University researchers had nine men perform cycling intervals, rest for 4 hours, then bike an endurance trial to exhaustion. At the beginning of the rest and again halfway through it, they drank either chocolate milk, a sports drink, or a carbohydrate-replacement drink. Those receiving chocolate milk or the sports drink cycled 54 percent longer than the men who relied on the carb-replacement drink. Study author Joel Stager, PhD, favors the flavored milk: "The chocolate contains antioxidants, and the milk has carbs, protein, and fat, plus micro- and macronutrients."

WEEK 10   WEEK OF / / TO / /   DAY:

STRENGTH TRAINING

| EXERCISE | WEIGHT | WARMUP SETS | | | WORK SETS | | |
		SET 1 REPS	SET 2 REPS	SET 3 REPS	SET 1 REPS	SET 2 REPS	SET 3 REPS

NOTES: _____

CARDIO

TYPE	INTENSITY	DURATION

NOTES: _____

TRAINING TIP
IS YOUR WORKOUT STALE?

Train smarter, not harder. In a 3-year study of 87 athletes, researchers at Indiana University in Bloomington found that nearly half had suffered from "staleness syndrome," a condition that causes exercise performance to plummet. The reason: Adhering to an intense workout routine for too long overwhelms your body, and training harder only makes it worse, says exercise psychologist and study author John Raglin, PhD. If the same workout suddenly becomes more difficult or you feel less enthused about exercising, you could be a victim. The fix: Allow your body to recover—cut the total repetitions that you normally perform in a workout by 50 percent for 1 to 2 weeks.

WEEK 11	WEEK OF / / TO / /	DAY:

STRENGTH TRAINING

EXERCISE	WEIGHT	WARMUP SETS			WORK SETS		
		SET 1 REPS	SET 2 REPS	SET 3 REPS	SET 1 REPS	SET 2 REPS	SET 3 REPS

NOTES:

CARDIO

TYPE	INTENSITY	DURATION

NOTES:

CORE POWER

SEATED AB CRUNCH

Sit on the edge of a bench. Grip the edge of the pad and lean back slightly, extending your legs down and away and keeping your heels 4 to 6 inches off the floor. Bend your knees and slowly raise your legs toward your chest.. At the same time, lean forward with your upper body, allowing your chest to approach your thighs. Return to the starting position. Perform three sets of 12 repetitions.

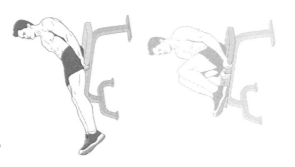

WEEK 11	WEEK OF / / TO / /	DAY:

STRENGTH TRAINING

EXERCISE	WEIGHT	WARM-UP SETS			WORK SETS		
		SET 1 REPS	SET 2 REPS	SET 3 REPS	SET 1 REPS	SET 2 REPS	SET 3 REPS

NOTES: _____

CARDIO

TYPE	INTENSITY	DURATION

NOTES: _____

FUELING UP

EGGS

Superpowers: builds muscle, burns fat

Secret weapons: protein, vitamin A, vitamin B

Fights against: obesity

HOW TO USE THEM

- Hard-boil a half-dozen eggs at a time for six any-time high-protein snacks.
- Eat them more often for breakfast. Whisk two eggs together in a microwaveable dish and cook them for 2 minutes, or until they're firmly set. Add some chopped vegetables—instant omelet.
- Add protein to your diet. Sneak eggs—particularly the omega-3-fortified kind—into other foods. They're a natural for beefing up stir-fries.

WEEK 11 | **WEEK OF / / TO / /** | **DAY:**

STRENGTH TRAINING

EXERCISE	WEIGHT	WARMUP SETS						WORK SETS					
		SET 1		SET 2		SET 3		SET 1		SET 2		SET 3	
		REPS		REPS		REPS		REPS		REPS		REPS	

NOTES:

CARDIO

TYPE	INTENSITY	DURATION

NOTES:

TRAINING TIP

EASY SET, HARD BODY

Add a light set to the end of your strength workout. In a study in the *Journal of Strength and Conditioning Research*, Japanese researchers found that your body will pump out more growth hormone if you finish your heavy-weight-lifting session with a single, high-repetition set of an exercise using light weight. "This could be partially responsible for greater strength gains," says Kazushige Goto, PhD, the study's lead author. A typical strength workout might be five reps at 90 percent of your one-rep max, followed by 20 reps at 50 percent of your one-rep max.

WEEK 11	WEEK OF / / TO / /	DAY:

STRENGTH TRAINING

EXERCISE	WEIGHT	WARMUP SETS			WORK SETS		
		SET 1 REPS	SET 2 REPS	SET 3 REPS	SET 1 REPS	SET 2 REPS	SET 3 REPS

NOTES: _____

CARDIO

TYPE	INTENSITY	DURATION

NOTES: _____

WEEK 12 WEEK OF / / TO / /   DAY:

STRENGTH TRAINING

EXERCISE	WEIGHT	WARMUP SETS			WORK SETS		
		SET 1 REPS	SET 2 REPS	SET 3 REPS	SET 1 REPS	SET 2 REPS	SET 3 REPS

NOTES: _____

CARDIO

TYPE	INTENSITY	DURATION

NOTES: _____

FUELING UP

SAY CHEESE

Cheese is a stellar source of calcium—and saturated fat. Is your favorite reduced-fat version truly as lean as the label suggests?

AMERICAN

Horizon Organic Reduced Fat, 60 calories, 2 grams saturated fat

Alpine Lace Reduced Fat, 90 calories, 5 grams saturated fat

CHEDDAR

Kerrygold Reduced Fat Vintage Irish, 70 calories, 3 grams saturated fat

Alpine Lace Reduced Fat, 90 calories, 5 grams saturated fat

MONTEREY JACK

Organic Valley Reduced Fat, 60 calories, 3 grams saturated fat

Tillamook Reduced Fat, 80 calories, 4 grams saturated fat

SPOTLIGHT EXERCISE

SWISS-BALL PUSHUP PLUS

Assume a pushup position with your hands placed directly under your shoulders and on the sides of a Swiss ball. Spread your fingers, with your thumbs pointing forward.

Keeping your core tight, lower yourself until your chest grazes the ball, then push back up. At the top of the move, push yourself as far away from the ball as you can so your shoulder blades move away from each other.

WEEK 12	WEEK OF / / TO / /	DAY:

STRENGTH TRAINING

		WARMUP SETS			WORK SETS		
		SET 1	SET 2	SET 3	SET 1	SET 2	SET 3
EXERCISE	WEIGHT	REPS	REPS	REPS	REPS	REPS	REPS

NOTES:

CARDIO

TYPE	INTENSITY	DURATION

NOTES:

WEEK 12 | WEEK OF / / TO / / | DAY:

STRENGTH TRAINING

EXERCISE	WEIGHT	WARMUP SETS			WORK SETS		
		SET 1 REPS	SET 2 REPS	SET 3 REPS	SET 1 REPS	SET 2 REPS	SET 3 REPS

NOTES: _____

CARDIO

TYPE	INTENSITY	DURATION

NOTES: _____

TRAINING TIP

CHEW THE FAT . . . AWAY

Lose your gut while you freshen your breath. British researchers found that chewing gum may help curb your cravings. When people chomped on sugarless gum for at least 15 minutes 1 hour after eating and then again at the 2-hour mark, their desire for sweets decreased by 11 percent compared with that of study participants who didn't work their jaws. The gum chewers also downed, on average, 36 fewer calories when they were turned loose on a buffet of sweet and salty snacks 3 hours after lunch. Although the researchers aren't sure why chewing sugarless gum helps, they suggest that because it exposes your tastebuds to sweetness, it could send a hunger-reducing signal to your brain. Interestingly, those who were the most calorie conscious experienced an even greater effect from the gum, says study author Marion Hetherington, PhD. Chomping on gum between meals reduced subsequent calorie intake by 8 percent.

FUELING UP

EAT ASPARAGUS NOW!

Peak season: March through June.

Sure, you can eat asparagus in December, but it probably will have traveled 5,000 miles before landing on your plate. Reality is, the spears will never be as tender or flavorful as they are in early Spring, when they're grown closer to home. Asparagus is loaded with bone-protecting vitamin K, and it's rich in folate, which may help ward off heart disease. "It's a nutritious alternative to starches as a side with fish or poultry," says Milton Stokes, MPH, RD, a spokesman for the American Dietetic Association. Toss a bunch with olive oil, cracked pepper, and Parmesan cheese. Roast for 10 minutes in a 400ºF oven or on a medium-high grill. Finish with a squeeze of lemon. When they're this fresh, they don't need much.

| WEEK 12 | WEEK OF / / TO / / | DAY: |

STRENGTH TRAINING

| | | WARMUP SETS | | | WORK SETS | | |
EXERCISE	WEIGHT	SET 1 REPS	SET 2 REPS	SET 3 REPS	SET 1 REPS	SET 2 REPS	SET 3 REPS

NOTES:

CARDIO

TYPE	INTENSITY	DURATION

NOTES:

SCULPT AND STRENGTHEN

PUSH HARDER FOR A SIX-PACK

Unleash your abs with the first exercise you ever learned, the pushup. Not just a chest builder, the pushup also strengthens your core, and it's a good indicator of whether or not you're exercising enough now to avoid the fat later. Canadian researchers found that guys who perform poorly in a pushup test are 78 percent more likely to gain 20 pounds of flab over the next 2 decades. Strive for 30 reps. "But don't stop there," says lead study author Peter Katzmarzyk, PhD. "The higher the number of pushups you can do, the lower your risk of weight gain," he says. And as a result, the better your abs.

WEEK 13 | WEEK OF / / TO / / | DAY:

STRENGTH TRAINING

EXERCISE	WEIGHT	WARMUP SETS			WORK SETS		
		SET 1 REPS	SET 2 REPS	SET 3 REPS	SET 1 REPS	SET 2 REPS	SET 3 REPS

NOTES:

CARDIO

TYPE	INTENSITY	DURATION

NOTES:

FITNESS FACT

WHY VEINS POP DURING EXERCISE

When you exercise, your heart beats faster and stronger, raising blood pressure. Arteries and veins are flooded with fast-flowing blood. The extra pressure in your blood vessels forces water out of your contracting muscles and into the compartments of muscle groups encased in fascia (strong connective tissue). The water causes the muscle compartments to swell and become dense and heavy. The swelling of the compartments pushes veins toward the skin's surface, so they appear to bulge. The veins remain there for about 30 minutes after exercise, when blood pressure drops and water returns to your muscles. Muscles are 80 percent water, but far less when in motion.

WEEK 13	WEEK OF / / TO / /	DAY:

STRENGTH TRAINING

EXERCISE	WEIGHT	WARMUP SETS			WORK SETS		
		SET 1 REPS	SET 2 REPS	SET 3 REPS	SET 1 REPS	SET 2 REPS	SET 3 REPS

NOTES:

CARDIO

TYPE	INTENSITY	DURATION

NOTES:

Ask the Trainer

How do I know when it's time to add weight?
—Victor, Lansing, MI

Make sure you can perform all your repetitions with your current weight for two consecutive workouts. Example: When you reach the upper limit of your repetition range with, say, 200 pounds—12 reps, maybe, if you're lifting to pack on size—make sure you perform 12 reps with 200 pounds during your next workout before adding more. And always add weight gradually: about 5 percent for each new step.

WEEK 13 | WEEK OF / / TO / / | DAY:

STRENGTH TRAINING

| EXERCISE | WEIGHT | WARM-UP SETS | | | WORK SETS | | |
		SET 1 REPS	SET 2 REPS	SET 3 REPS	SET 1 REPS	SET 2 REPS	SET 3 REPS

NOTES:

CARDIO

TYPE	INTENSITY	DURATION

NOTES:

FITNESS FACT

STAY STRONG

Great news for men hard-pressed for time: Researchers at the University of New Brunswick, in Canada, found that seasoned lifters can maintain strength with one workout a week. In the study, men who stopped working out for 9 weeks lost significant amounts of strength, while those who reduced their training from 3 days a week to once a week maintained their strength. "Over that short period of time, once per week appears adequate to maintain strength," says study author James Sexsmith, PhD.

WEEK 13 | **WEEK OF / / TO / /** | **DAY:**

STRENGTH TRAINING

EXERCISE	WEIGHT	WARMUP SETS						WORK SETS					
		SET 1		SET 2		SET 3		SET 1		SET 2		SET 3	
		REPS		REPS		REPS		REPS		REPS		REPS	

NOTES: _____

CARDIO

TYPE	INTENSITY	DURATION

NOTES: _____

FUELING UP

FUEL THE BURN

Start your meal with something spicy. Researchers in the Netherlands found that eating hot peppers may help you eat less. In the study, 12 men ate 0.9 gram of ground chile peppers—in pill form or mixed into a tomato-juice beverage—30 minutes before getting a free run at an all-you-can-eat buffet. Compared with a placebo, the pill helped men cut their food intakes by 10 percent, while the liquid mixture resulted in a 16 percent reduction. The pepper-primed eaters chose fewer calorie-dense foods, says study author Margriet Westerterp, PhD. Get your meal off to a searing start with an extra-spicy Bloody Mary or a cup of chili spiked with Tabasco.

WEEK 14 **WEEK OF / / TO / /** **DAY:**

STRENGTH TRAINING

EXERCISE	WEIGHT	WARMUP SETS			WORK SETS		
		SET 1 REPS	SET 2 REPS	SET 3 REPS	SET 1 REPS	SET 2 REPS	SET 3 REPS

NOTES:

CARDIO

TYPE	INTENSITY	DURATION

NOTES:

TRAINING TIP
THE BEST START

Overweight men trying to improve their cardiovascular health should be more concerned with the amount of exercise they do and not its intensity, according to a study in the journal *Chest*. Duke researchers working with 133 people for 9 months found that among unfit overweight people, increasing the amount of exercise leads to significant improvements in fitness, while raising intensity doesn't. Later on, "as fitness increases, intensity becomes important," says study author Brian Duscha. If you're a beginner, Duscha recommends jogging or walking 12 miles a week at 40 to 55 percent of your peak heart rate. Then, for the best gains, kick it up to 20 miles a week at the same intensity.

WEEK 14 | WEEK OF / / TO / / | DAY:

STRENGTH TRAINING

EXERCISE	WEIGHT	WARMUP SETS			WORK SETS		
		SET 1 REPS	SET 2 REPS	SET 3 REPS	SET 1 REPS	SET 2 REPS	SET 3 REPS

NOTES:

CARDIO

TYPE	INTENSITY	DURATION

NOTES:

FUELING UP

RASPBERRIES AND OTHER BERRIES

Secret weapons: antioxidants (including vitamin C), fiber, tannins (in cranberries)

Fights against: heart disease, cancer, obesity

HOW TO USE THEM

- Blend them into a smoothie. Fresh or frozen berries can go straight in; frozen berries will add a rich, creamy texture to the mix.
- Add them to instant oatmeal. Toss some frozen berries into uncooked oatmeal, pour boiling water on top, and mix gently. You'll have a fast breakfast.
- Sprinkle them in plain or vanilla yogurt.

Berry Wafflewich

1   whole wheat toaster waffle

½   tablespoon peanut butter

¼   cup slightly crushed blueberries, blackberries, or raspberries

Prepare the waffle according to the package directions. Spread the peanut butter on the waffle. Cup the waffle in your hand, add the berries, then squeeze lightly. Think of it as a berry breakfast taco.

WEEK 14   WEEK OF / / TO / /   DAY:

STRENGTH TRAINING

EXERCISE	WEIGHT	WARMUP SETS SET 1 REPS	SET 2 REPS	SET 3 REPS	WORK SETS SET 1 REPS	SET 2 REPS	SET 3 REPS

NOTES: _____

CARDIO

TYPE	INTENSITY	DURATION

NOTES: _____

HOOK UP AT THE CABLE STATION

Don't know how to break the ice with that gym babe? "I would be totally impressed if a man asked for help on how to do an exercise," says Dana DiPasquale, an exercise physiologist. "Macho, know-it-all guys are a definite turnoff. Stupid guys are turnoffs too, so don't ask how to jump rope.

WEEK 14 | WEEK OF / / TO / / | DAY: _____

STRENGTH TRAINING

EXERCISE	WEIGHT	WARMUP SETS						WORK SETS		
		SET 1 REPS	SET 2 REPS	SET 3 REPS	SET 1 REPS	SET 2 REPS	SET 3 REPS	SET 1 REPS	SET 2 REPS	SET 3 REPS

NOTES: _____

CARDIO

TYPE	INTENSITY	DURATION

NOTES: _____

83

TRAINING TIP

THE GOLDEN ARCH

Don't bend over backward for your workout. According to a report published in the *Strength and Conditioning Journal*, your lower back is most susceptible to injury when it's either fully flexed or fully extended. The advice is simple: "When you lift weights, keep a natural arch in your spine," says Robert Manske, CSCS, coauthor of the report. "Most back injuries are strains or sprains, which stem from poor lifting form or fatigue." For nearly every exercise—situps and back extensions excluded—your lower back should maintain the form it has when you're standing with good posture. Use a mirror as a reference.

WEEK 15	WEEK OF / / TO / /	DAY:

STRENGTH TRAINING

		WARMUP SETS						WORK SETS					
EXERCISE	WEIGHT	SET 1		SET 2		SET 3		SET 1		SET 2		SET 3	
		REPS		REPS		REPS		REPS		REPS		REPS	

NOTES:

CARDIO

TYPE	INTENSITY	DURATION

NOTES:

Ask the Trainer

How can I bench at home without a spotter?
—Seth, Oxnard, CA

We've all heard horror stories of men being pinned under more weight than they could handle. One solution is to do a variation on the "rest pause" principle. With rest pause, you end up handling more weight than you ordinarily could, by taking short breaks during a set. Here's how it works.

Select a weight that normally allows you to perform only four or five repetitions (without going to absolute failure). After doing four or five reps, pause and rack the weight for 10 seconds.

Next, grab the bar and crank out whatever you can safely do (usually about another one or two reps) before racking the weight again. This time, rest for 15 to 20 seconds, and then try for another couple of repetitions.

Rack the weight one last time and rest for 20 to 30 seconds before grinding out one or two more. By the time you're finished, you should have amassed anywhere from 8 to 12 repetitions with a weight that ordinarily allows you to do only 4 or 5. The end result is more size and strength, and a windpipe that remains intact.

WEEK 15 | **WEEK OF / / TO / /** | **DAY:** ___

STRENGTH TRAINING

EXERCISE	WEIGHT	WARMUP SETS			WORK SETS		
		SET 1 REPS	SET 2 REPS	SET 3 REPS	SET 1 REPS	SET 2 REPS	SET 3 REPS

NOTES: _____

CARDIO

TYPE	INTENSITY	DURATION

NOTES: _____

STRETCH IT OUT

PREPARE FOR YOUR BACK ROUTINE

TOUCHDOWN

1. Stand with your arms at your sides. Keep your arms straight and your abs and glutes tight.

2. Raise your arms in front of you in an arc until they're behind your head and slightly out to the sides. Perform 15 to 20 reps.

SCAPULAR PUSHUP

1. Put your hands directly under your shoulders on a Swiss ball.

2. With arms slightly bent, pinch your shoulder blades together for 2 seconds, then push them apart and pause. Do 12 to 15 reps.

WEEK 15 | **WEEK OF / / TO / /** | **DAY:**

STRENGTH TRAINING

EXERCISE	WEIGHT	WARMUP SETS						WORK SETS					
		SET 1		SET 2		SET 3		SET 1		SET 2		SET 3	
		REPS		REPS		REPS		REPS		REPS		REPS	

NOTES: _____

CARDIO

TYPE	INTENSITY	DURATION

NOTES: _____

BIG LIES

Just because an exercise looks cool doesn't mean it works. "Many weight-room beliefs are based on anecdotal evidence," says Michael Bird, PhD, of Truman State University in Kirksville, Missouri. Dr. Bird tested one such belief: that rotating your foot for standing calf raises emphasizes different portions of the gastrocnemius, the most visible calf muscle. His study found that angling your feet inward or outward does not work calf muscles any differently than keeping your toes pointed straight ahead. Try the seated calf raise as a better variation.

WEEK 15 | WEEK OF / / TO / / | DAY:

STRENGTH TRAINING

EXERCISE	WEIGHT	WARMUP SETS			WORK SETS		
		SET 1 REPS	SET 2 REPS	SET 3 REPS	SET 1 REPS	SET 2 REPS	SET 3 REPS

NOTES:

CARDIO

TYPE	INTENSITY	DURATION

NOTES:

TRAINING TIP
GROWING PAINS

Soreness may not be the best indicator of whether or not to repeat a workout. Researchers in Taiwan found that performing heavy biceps curls with sore muscles didn't slow recovery from a bout of exercise 3 days earlier. And although soreness can linger for several days after you lift, previous research has shown that muscles grow for just 48 hours after a training session. This suggests that working each muscle group every other day is the best way to build size, regardless of how sore you might be. One caveat: If you notice that you don't perform as well from one workout to the next—for instance, you can't complete at least as many sets and repetitions with the same weight—consider it a sign that your muscles need an additional day or two of rest, says lead researcher Trevor Chen, PhD.

WEEK 16 | **WEEK OF / / TO / /** | **DAY:**

STRENGTH TRAINING

EXERCISE	WEIGHT	WARMUP SETS						WORK SETS					
		SET 1		SET 2		SET 3		SET 1		SET 2		SET 3	
		REPS		REPS		REPS		REPS		REPS		REPS	

NOTES: _____

CARDIO

TYPE	INTENSITY	DURATION

NOTES: _____

SPOTLIGHT EXERCISE

SIDE JACKKNIFE

Lie on your left side with your torso propped up on your left forearm and your legs nearly straight. Hold your right hand behind your right ear, with your elbow pointed toward your feet. While keeping your torso stationary, lift your legs as far as you can. The motion should feel like a crunch—a contraction on the right side of your waist and in your core. Slowly lower your legs and repeat. Finish a set of 10 repetitions on that side, then flip to your right side and do another 10. Switch back and forth for a total of three sets on each side.

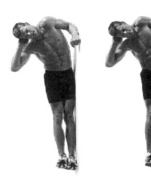

WEEK 16 | WEEK OF / / TO / / | DAY:

STRENGTH TRAINING

EXERCISE	WEIGHT	WARMUP SETS			WORK SETS		
		SET 1 REPS	SET 2 REPS	SET 3 REPS	SET 1 REPS	SET 2 REPS	SET 3 REPS

NOTES:

CARDIO

TYPE	INTENSITY	DURATION

NOTES:

Ask the Trainer

Lots of diets say you can eat whatever you want 1 day a week. So can I have a few bad things, or can I totally binge?

—*Mark, Skokie, IL*

Weight isn't the only issue here. It takes a 3,500-calorie surplus to pack on 1 pound, so you'd have to chow down to notice an effect. The real worry is that even one high-fat, high-carbohydrate load can boost oxidative stress in the body and make it harder to resist new temptations. The bottom line: Cheating on your diet doesn't mean abandoning it entirely. Limit your splurge to a few forbidden snacks.

WEEK 16 **WEEK OF** / / **TO** / / **DAY:**

STRENGTH TRAINING

EXERCISE	WEIGHT	WARMUP SETS SET 1 REPS	SET 2 REPS	SET 3 REPS	WORK SETS SET 1 REPS	SET 2 REPS	SET 3 REPS

NOTES:

CARDIO

TYPE	INTENSITY	DURATION

NOTES:

TRAINING TIP
WHEN SECONDS COUNT

A longer workout doesn't always mean a better one. According to a recent report published in the *Strength and Conditioning Journal*, men often take up to 90 minutes to complete a workout that should take just 45. The likely reason? Resting too long after each set, says *Men's Health* Muscle Guy Mike Mejia, CSCS. Keep an eye on the clock: Studies show that taking 60 to 75 seconds of recovery time between sets is a highly effective strategy for both building muscle and losing fat. But if you're mainly interested in boosting strength, resting longer between sets works best.

WEEK 16	WEEK OF / / TO / /	DAY:

STRENGTH TRAINING

EXERCISE	WEIGHT	WARMUP SETS			WORK SETS		
		SET 1 REPS	SET 2 REPS	SET 3 REPS	SET 1 REPS	SET 2 REPS	SET 3 REPS

NOTES: _____

CARDIO

TYPE	INTENSITY	DURATION

NOTES: _____

SCULPT AND STRENGTHEN

THE EXTRA-STRENGTH FORMULA

Make boosting your bench press a guessing game—for your muscles. Varying your reps and resistance every workout can double your strength gains compared with a more conventional approach in which you mix it up every few weeks, report researchers at Arizona State University. "More-frequent changes appear to better stimulate the neuromuscular system, which is largely responsible for strength gains," says Mark Peterson, CSCS. Do three sets of 10 reps of each exercise on Monday, two sets of 15 on Wednesday, and four sets of 5 on Friday. Adjust the amount of weight you lift each day, so your muscles are always challenged.

WEEK 17 | WEEK OF / / TO / / | DAY:

STRENGTH TRAINING

EXERCISE	WEIGHT	WARMUP SETS						WORK SETS					
		SET 1		SET 2		SET 3		SET 1		SET 2		SET 3	
		REPS		REPS		REPS		REPS		REPS		REPS	

NOTES:

CARDIO

TYPE	INTENSITY	DURATION

NOTES:

LIFT TODAY, RUN TOMORROW

Weight-lifting newbies don't have to worry that cardio work will limit their strength gains. Researchers at Texas A&M University studied 31 men (all new to weight lifting) in three groups over 12 weeks. Some did only resistance training, some did only endurance training, and some did both. Those who did both types of training and those who only lifted weights improved strength equally, by 40 percent. "Beginners see huge strength gains in the first 4 to 6 weeks, due to neurological changes," says lead study author Shawn Glowacki, PhD. But, for best results, do cardio and strength training on alternate days so they don't interfere with each other.

WEEK 17 | **WEEK OF / / TO / /** | **DAY:**

STRENGTH TRAINING

EXERCISE	WEIGHT	WARMUP SETS			WORK SETS		
		SET 1 REPS	SET 2 REPS	SET 3 REPS	SET 1 REPS	SET 2 REPS	SET 3 REPS

NOTES: _____

CARDIO

TYPE	INTENSITY	DURATION

NOTES: _____

Ask the Trainer

Does it matter if I lift weights in running shoes?
—*Ted, Newark, DE*

Does it matter if you run a marathon in Timberlands? "If you're doing standing exercises or anything with lateral movements (such as side lunges), running shoes can make you susceptible to injury," says Stephen Pribut, DPM, president of the American Academy of Podiatric Sports Medicine. They have extra cushioning, which can affect your balance. It's like standing on a foam cushion versus a hard floor, says Dr. Pribut. Cross-trainers and tennis shoes have flatter soles," says Dr. Pribut, "and provide better support for lifting."

A flat-soled sneaker gives weight lifters the stability they need.

The elevated heel of a running shoe makes it ill-suited for a weight-lifting session.

WEEK 17	WEEK OF / / TO / /	DAY:

STRENGTH TRAINING

EXERCISE	WEIGHT	WARMUP SETS			WORK SETS		
		SET 1 REPS	SET 2 REPS	SET 3 REPS	SET 1 REPS	SET 2 REPS	SET 3 REPS

NOTES:

CARDIO

TYPE	INTENSITY	DURATION

NOTES:

SCULPT AND STRENGTHEN

PRACTICAL STRENGTH

This plan yields bulk and core strength. Perform three circuits, resting for 2 minutes after each.

DUMBBELL DEADLIFT

Stand with a heavy dumbbell on the floor beside each foot. Bend your knees and grab the weights with your palms facing in. Keeping your head and chest up, your back arched, and your torso forward no more than 45 degrees, stand up. Then lower yourself, maintaining the arch in your back.

FLOOR PRESS

Lie down with your knees bent, feet on the floor and your upper arms in contact with the floor. Hold a pair of heavy dumbbells next to your shoulders, as if you were about to perform a bench press. Press the weights up over your chest, then lower them.

NEGATIVE SITUP

Sit on the floor with your knees bent 90 degrees and hold a dumbbell with both hands close to your chest. Take 5 or 6 seconds to lower your back toward the floor, one vertebra at a time. Sit back up using as little momentum as possible.

WEEK 17 | **WEEK OF** / / **TO** / / | **DAY:**

STRENGTH TRAINING

EXERCISE	WEIGHT	WARMUP SETS			WORK SETS		
		SET 1 REPS	SET 2 REPS	SET 3 REPS	SET 1 REPS	SET 2 REPS	SET 3 REPS

NOTES: _____

CARDIO

TYPE	INTENSITY	DURATION

NOTES: _____

FUELING UP
MOO FOR YOUR MIDSECTION

The Dow might be bearish, but we predict a bull market for dairy producers. Research at the University of Tennessee found that eating yogurt can help you lose weight and zap the flab from your gut. In the 12-week study, people who consumed three 6-ounce servings of fat-free yogurt daily lost 81 percent more fat from their midsections than those who ate a variety of dairy products containing less total calcium. The mineral appears to help curb production of the stress hormone cortisol, which has been linked to the accumulation of abdominal fat, says lead researcher Michael Zemel, PhD. Our favorite fat-free yogurt: Stonyfield Farm.

WEEK 18	WEEK OF / / TO / /	DAY:

STRENGTH TRAINING

EXERCISE	WEIGHT	WARMUP SETS			WORK SETS		
		SET 1 REPS	SET 2 REPS	SET 3 REPS	SET 1 REPS	SET 2 REPS	SET 3 REPS

NOTES: _____

CARDIO

TYPE	INTENSITY	DURATION

NOTES: _____

FITNESS FACT
MIND-BODY CONNECTION

It really is all in your head: U.K. researchers found that men bench-press 12 percent more weight when they psych themselves up before a lift than when they're distracted. In the study, the scientists either gave experienced weight lifters 20 seconds to prepare mentally for three sets of five repetitions of a strength exercise or asked them to count backward from 1,000 in increments of seven before the sets. The take-home message: Before you approach the bench, skip the small talk and focus on the task at hand.

WEEK 18 | WEEK OF / / TO / / | DAY:

STRENGTH TRAINING

EXERCISE	WEIGHT	WARMUP SETS						WORK SETS					
		SET 1		SET 2		SET 3		SET 1		SET 2		SET 3	
		REPS		REPS		REPS		REPS		REPS		REPS	

NOTES:

CARDIO

TYPE	INTENSITY	DURATION

NOTES:

CORE POWER

KNEE RAISE WITH DROP

Lie on your back with your hands behind your ears, your feet on the floor, and a medicine ball held between bent knees. Keeping your lower back on the floor, contract your abdominals and pull your knees toward your chest. Lower your knees to the left, bring them back to the center, then return to the starting position. On the next repetition, drop your knees to the right, and alternate sides for each rep. Do three sets of 12 repetitions.

WEEK 18	WEEK OF / / TO / /	DAY:

STRENGTH TRAINING

	WEIGHT	WARMUP SETS			WORK SETS		
EXERCISE		SET 1 REPS	SET 2 REPS	SET 3 REPS	SET 1 REPS	SET 2 REPS	SET 3 REPS

NOTES:

CARDIO

TYPE	INTENSITY	DURATION

NOTES:

FUELING UP

FILL YOURSELF WITH FIBER

New research has identified another way fiber can help you drop pounds. In a study at the University of Tromsø in Norway, 176 overweight people who followed a reduced-calorie diet and took daily fiber supplements for a month lost nearly twice as much weight as people on the same low-calorie diet who popped a placebo. The supplemental fiber—4 grams daily—performed the same trick as fiber from food: It made them feel full, so they ended up eating less. But don't load up on Metamucil. Although three brands of supplements were used in the study, researchers credit their common ingredient: glucomannan, a type of soluble dietary fiber derived from tubers of the *Amorphophallus konjac* plant. It's sold in powder and caplet forms at vitamin stores.

WEEK 18 | WEEK OF / / TO / / | DAY:

STRENGTH TRAINING

EXERCISE	WEIGHT	WARMUP SETS			WORK SETS		
		SET 1 REPS	SET 2 REPS	SET 3 REPS	SET 1 REPS	SET 2 REPS	SET 3 REPS

NOTES:

CARDIO

TYPE	INTENSITY	DURATION

NOTES:

BODY MOVING

RISE AND WALK

Think twice about skipping workouts. Researchers at the University of Missouri at Columbia have found that your muscles' insulin efficiency decreases after just 2 days of inactivity. A drop in insulin efficiency can increase your chances of developing diabetes, high blood pressure, and heart disease. Study author Frank Booth, PhD, a professor of biomedical sciences, says that after rest, receptors on muscle cells "become less efficient at signaling the amount of insulin bound to them," and less glucose is taken into your muscles for energy. That leaves more glucose to wreak havoc in the rest of your body. Booth suggests physical activity most days of the week (walking is good), especially if type 2 diabetes runs in your family.

WEEK 19	WEEK OF / / TO / /	DAY:

STRENGTH TRAINING

EXERCISE	WEIGHT	WARMUP SETS			WORK SETS		
		SET 1	SET 2	SET 3	SET 1	SET 2	SET 3
		REPS	REPS	REPS	REPS	REPS	REPS

NOTES: _____

CARDIO

TYPE	INTENSITY	DURATION

NOTES: _____

TRAINING TIP

DO FEWER SETS FOR A BIGGER CHEST

In a study published in the *Journal of Sports Medicine and Physical Fitness*, men who did fewer sets of bench presses with longer rest periods in between gained nearly twice as much strength as men who did more sets with shorter rest periods. Lifting the same amount of weight, the men did either four sets of six repetitions with 65 seconds of rest between sets, or eight sets of three reps with 14 seconds of rest between sets. Fewer sets and longer rest periods "would appear superior for strength gains," says John Cronin, PhD, the lead study author.

| WEEK 19 | WEEK OF / / TO / / | DAY: |

STRENGTH TRAINING

EXERCISE	WEIGHT	WARMUP SETS						WORK SETS					
		SET 1		SET 2		SET 3		SET 1		SET 2		SET 3	
		REPS		REPS		REPS		REPS		REPS		REPS	

NOTES: _____

CARDIO

TYPE	INTENSITY	DURATION

NOTES: _____

STRETCH IT OUT

GET A POWERFUL WARMUP

A Japanese study in the *Journal of Strength and Conditioning Research* found that static stretching has no positive effect on muscular performance. Eleven men who performed five lower-body static stretches (slowly stretching and holding for 30 seconds) showed decreased leg power afterward. When the same men did dynamic stretches (involving movement and contraction of the muscle that's opposite the one targeted), leg power increased by 10 percent. Greater muscle-activity level and temperature increase probably caused the improvement, says study author Taichi Yamaguchi, MS, chair of health and sports science at Hokkaido University in Sapporo.

WEEK 19 WEEK OF / / TO / / DAY:

STRENGTH TRAINING

EXERCISE	WEIGHT	WARMUP SETS			WORK SETS		
		SET 1 REPS	SET 2 REPS	SET 3 REPS	SET 1 REPS	SET 2 REPS	SET 3 REPS

NOTES:

CARDIO

TYPE	INTENSITY	DURATION

NOTES:

Ask the Trainer

I slouch. How can I straighten my shoulders?
—Chris, Memphis

Perform the following exercises as one set:

1. **Split-stance rotation.** Kneel on one knee and hold a broom or golf club across your shoulders with your hands shoulder-width apart. Rotate your upper back toward your raised knee by turning your shoulders as far as you can. Pause for two seconds. Do 10 repetitions on each side.

2. **Single-arm face pull.** With your left hand, grab a rope handle and attach it to a high-pulley cable, standing an arm's length away. Pull your shoulder blades back and down. Then, bending from your elbow, pull the handle alongside your head until it passes your left ear. Do 15 reps with each arm.

WEEK 19 | WEEK OF / / TO / / | DAY:

STRENGTH TRAINING

EXERCISE	WEIGHT	WARMUP SETS			WORK SETS		
		SET 1 REPS	SET 2 REPS	SET 3 REPS	SET 1 REPS	SET 2 REPS	SET 3 REPS

NOTES: _____

CARDIO

TYPE	INTENSITY	DURATION

NOTES: _____

103

STRETCH IT OUT

THE NEW WARMUP: EAGLE STRETCH

Stretch your hips, groin, and hamstrings with this move from Blair O'Donovan, CSCS, sports-conditioning director at Elite Athlete Training Systems, in Maryland.

Stand with your feet slightly more than shoulder-width apart. Keeping your back naturally arched, bend at the hips and knees to lower your body. Hold the bottom position for 2 seconds while you use your elbows to push your knees away from each other, promoting a deeper stretch through your hips and groin. Return to the starting position and repeat 10 to 12 times.

WEEK 20   WEEK OF / / TO / /   DAY:

STRENGTH TRAINING

EXERCISE	WEIGHT	WARMUP SETS			WORK SETS		
		SET 1 REPS	SET 2 REPS	SET 3 REPS	SET 1 REPS	SET 2 REPS	SET 3 REPS

NOTES: _____

CARDIO

TYPE	INTENSITY	DURATION

NOTES: _____

TRAINING TIP

HIP AT THE NEXT LEVEL

Strengthening your hips can help your hops. A study published in the *Journal of Strength and Conditioning Research* found that your hip-extensor muscles—mainly the hamstrings and gluteus maximus—are more responsible for your ability to jump high than are your calves, quads, or ankles. The researchers measured the amount of muscle activity at the ankle, knee, and hip joints when men jumped low and when they jumped high. Activity levels remained the same at the ankles and knees for low jumps and high jumps, but were greater at the hip for the highest jumps, says lead author Adrian Lees, PhD. Target your hamstrings and glutes with squats, hamstring curls, and glute bridges.

WEEK 20	WEEK OF / / TO / /	DAY:

STRENGTH TRAINING

EXERCISE	WEIGHT	WARM UP SETS			WORK SETS		
		SET 1 REPS	SET 2 REPS	SET 3 REPS	SET 1 REPS	SET 2 REPS	SET 3 REPS

NOTES: _____

CARDIO

TYPE	INTENSITY	DURATION

NOTES: _____

CORE POWER

HOW TO AVOID A KILLER GUT

Hit the road to see your abs: Burning 1,100 calories a week through exercise prevents the accumulation of dangerous belly fat. In a new 6-month study, Duke University scientists tracked 175 people's levels of visceral adipose tissue—the type of abdominal flab that causes high blood sugar, hypertension, and arterial inflammation. Those who walked or jogged at least 11 miles a week didn't gain any of the deadly fat—regardless of their exercise intensity or diet—while the nonexercisers increased their belly-fat stores by 9 percent. If you're not into walking 11 miles, you can burn 1,100 calories in a week by cycling 22 miles, swimming for 102 minutes, or performing three 30-minute circuit-training workouts. Not happy with just maintaining? Crank it up a bit; men who burned an additional 550 calories reduced their visceral-fat levels by 7 percent.

WEEK 20 | WEEK OF / / TO / / | DAY:

STRENGTH TRAINING

EXERCISE	WEIGHT	WARMUP SETS			WORK SETS		
		SET 1 REPS	SET 2 REPS	SET 3 REPS	SET 1 REPS	SET 2 REPS	SET 3 REPS

NOTES: _____

CARDIO

TYPE	INTENSITY	DURATION

NOTES: _____

FITNESS FACT

SCARE YOURSELF SLIM

Now there's research behind the Nike slogan "Just Do It." Successful exercisers don't think about having to train, they just get out there, says Sandra Cousins, EdD, an exercise gerontologist at the University of Alberta in Edmonton. After conducting 40 interviews, she found that people who relied on self pep talks to motivate themselves to exercise remained inactive. "They are simply not ready," she says. Need a jump start? According to a study in the *Journal of Sport and Exercise Physiology*, writing about your mortality can boost motivation. Write down how the thought of your own death makes you feel, and read it in the morning. That should get you moving.

WEEK 20	WEEK OF / / TO / /	DAY:

STRENGTH TRAINING

EXERCISE	WEIGHT	WARMUP SETS			WORK SETS		
		SET 1	SET 2	SET 3	SET 1	SET 2	SET 3
		REPS	REPS	REPS	REPS	REPS	REPS

NOTES:

CARDIO

TYPE	INTENSITY	DURATION

NOTES:

Ask the Trainer

My back kills me at my desk. What can I do?
—Vance, Shaker Heights, OH

Bill Hartman, PT, CSCS suggests:

HIP FLEXOR

Kneel on your right knee, tighten your right buttock, reach up with your right arm, and bend to the left. Do this to each side at least once for 20 seconds. "This counteracts the position of sitting, because it's the opposite activity—instead of having your hip bent, it's extended," Hartman says.

GLUTE BRIDGE

Lie on your back with your knees bent, squeeze your buttocks together, and lift your hips off the floor. Hold for 5 seconds and repeat 12 times. "By contracting the buttocks, you're stretching the front side of the hip," Hartman says.

WEEK 21 | WEEK OF / / TO / / | DAY:

STRENGTH TRAINING

EXERCISE	WEIGHT	WARMUP SETS						WORK SETS					
		SET 1		SET 2		SET 3		SET 1		SET 2		SET 3	
		REPS		REPS		REPS		REPS		REPS		REPS	

NOTES:

CARDIO

TYPE	INTENSITY	DURATION

NOTES:

FIVE GOLDEN RULES OF THE GYM

We asked guys about their workout habits in a recent online poll, and came up with this set of unwritten workout laws.

Don't leave DNA behind

35: Percentage of guys who fail to wipe down machines after using them

Don't go big without a spotter

23: Percentage of men who have been pinned by a loaded barbell

Maintain proper order

16: Percentage of guys who don't return dumbbells to their rightful spot

Stay off girly machines

30: Percentage of men who use the inner- and outer-thigh machines

Follow the "urinal rule"

65: Percentage of guys who opt for the machine next to someone when others are open

---

WEEK 21 | WEEK OF / / TO / / | DAY:

STRENGTH TRAINING

EXERCISE	WEIGHT	WARMUP SETS SET1 REPS	WARMUP SETS SET2 REPS	WARMUP SETS SET3 REPS	WORK SETS SET1 REPS	WORK SETS SET2 REPS	WORK SETS SET3 REPS

NOTES:

CARDIO

TYPE	INTENSITY	DURATION

NOTES:

FITNESS FACT

POUND ADVICE

Take a load off; you'll feel better. Scientists at Wake Forest University found that for every pound of weight you lose, you alleviate the pressure on your knees by 4 pounds. In addition to reducing joint pain, weight loss may also improve range of motion and reduce the demand on nearby muscles to provide stability, says Stephen Messier, PhD, the study author. If knee troubles are keeping you from exercising in the first place, try rowing instead of running. Or walk on an inclined treadmill; it allows you to exert your highest effort without forcing you to break into a joint-pounding jog.

WEEK OF / / TO / /   DAY:

STRENGTH TRAINING

EXERCISE	WEIGHT	WARMUP SETS						WORK SETS					
		SET 1		SET 2		SET 3		SET 1		SET 2		SET 3	
		REPS		REPS		REPS		REPS		REPS		REPS	

NOTES:

CARDIO

TYPE	INTENSITY	DURATION

NOTES:

FUELING UP
NO BANG FROM YOUR STARBUCKS

Don't count on a caffeine lift at the gym, says a University of Nebraska study. During an 8-week endurance-training program, exercisers on decaf experienced the same fitness gains as daily caffeine users. Eighteen college students downed a 200-milligram caffeine pill an hour before three weekly workouts and took the supplement before breakfast on days off. Eighteen others took a placebo and trained on the same schedule. After the 8 weeks, time to exhaustion and body composition were equal in both groups. Apparently, the caffeinated exercisers adjusted to the stimulant, so there was no performance effect, says study author Moh Malek, CSCS.

WEEK 21 WEEK OF / / TO / /   DAY:

STRENGTH TRAINING

EXERCISE	WEIGHT	WARMUP SETS			WORK SETS		
		SET 1 REPS	SET 2 REPS	SET 3 REPS	SET 1 REPS	SET 2 REPS	SET 3 REPS

NOTES:

CARDIO

TYPE	INTENSITY	DURATION

NOTES:

WEEK 22	WEEK OF / / TO / /	DAY:

SPOTLIGHT EXERCISE

JUMP-START YOUR GAME

Take your squat—and your results—to new heights. Researchers at the College of New Jersey recently discovered that adding a jump squat to your workout can boost strength by as much as 13 percent in 5 weeks. In the study, men who did jump squats twice a week during the last third of a 15-week program improved their standard barbell squats by an average of 66 pounds. "The jump squat trains your muscles for explosive power, a stimulus for gains that traditional lifting doesn't provide," says lead study author Jay Hoffman, PhD. Try adding the move to your routine.

JUMP SQUAT

Hold a light barbell with an overhand grip so that it rests comfortably on your upper back (not on your neck). Set your feet shoulder-width apart, with your knees slightly bent, your back straight, and your eyes focused straight ahead. Slowly lower your body as if you were sitting back into a chair, keeping your back in its natural alignment and your lower legs nearly perpendicular to the floor. When your thighs are parallel to the floor, push off forcefully to jump up as high as you can. Sink directly into the next squat without pausing.

STRENGTH TRAINING

EXERCISE	WEIGHT	WARMUP SETS			WORK SETS		
		SET 1 REPS	SET 2 REPS	SET 3 REPS	SET 1 REPS	SET 2 REPS	SET 3 REPS

NOTES: _____

CARDIO

TYPE	INTENSITY	DURATION

NOTES: _____

SHOULDER NO LOAD

Get strong without weights. Two Swiss balls can pump up your shoulders in no time. Try this shoulder-press variation from Mike Mejia, MS, CSCS.

Position two small Swiss balls together and lie back on them so that your head is between, but not resting, on them. Your upper back and shoulders should rest on the balls. Keep your knees bent and your hips raised so your body looks like a table. Bend your elbows 90 degrees.

With your abs tight, straighten one arm over your head. (Try to keep that shoulder in contact with the ball.) Bring your arm back down, then straighten your other arm. "Both shoulders, especially the shoulder of the straight arm, have to work hard to stabilize you," says Mejia. Try for two sets of 8 to 10 reps.

WEEK 22 | WEEK OF / / TO / / | DAY:

STRENGTH TRAINING

EXERCISE	WEIGHT	WARMUP SETS			WORK SETS		
		SET 1 REPS	SET 2 REPS	SET 3 REPS	SET 1 REPS	SET 2 REPS	SET 3 REPS

NOTES: _____

CARDIO

TYPE	INTENSITY	DURATION

NOTES: _____

WEEK OF / / TO / / DAY:

FUELING UP

Tropical Smoothie

½ cup 1% milk
2 tablespoons low-fat yogurt
¼ cup frozen orange-juice concentrate
½ banana
¼ cup strawberries
½ cup cubed mango
2 teaspoons vanilla whey-protein powder
3 ice cubes

Chuck everything into a blender. Crank it.

STRENGTH TRAINING

EXERCISE	WEIGHT	WARMUP SETS			WORK SETS		
		SET 1 REPS	SET 2 REPS	SET 3 REPS	SET 1 REPS	SET 2 REPS	SET 3 REPS

NOTES:

CARDIO

TYPE	INTENSITY	DURATION

NOTES:

TRAINING TIP

PUSHUP TRICKS

Hit your chest from every angle with these pushups from strength coach Scott Rankin, CSCS.

Standard: Place your hands directly beneath your shoulders. Keep your abs tight and your body in a straight line from ear to ankle. This activates pecs more deeply than variations do.

Narrow-Base: Place your hands less than shoulder-width apart. Keep your elbows out and squeeze your pecs together at the top of the move. Activating the medial portion of the pectorals (close to the sternum) helps define your inner chest to create a separation.

Wide-Base: Place your hands more than shoulder-width apart. This variation increases the stretch on the pectorals, which helps develop the outer portion of your chest.

Decline: Place your toes on a bench or Swiss ball to stress your lower chest. Your shoulders work even harder to stabilize you.

Incline: Place your hands on a bench. It's easier, so it's a good way to completely fatigue your chest after you've done as many reps as you can of the standard version.

WEEK 22 | WEEK OF / / TO / / | DAY:

STRENGTH TRAINING

EXERCISE	WEIGHT	WARMUP SETS			WORK SETS		
		SET 1 REPS	SET 2 REPS	SET 3 REPS	SET 1 REPS	SET 2 REPS	SET 3 REPS

NOTES:

CARDIO

TYPE	INTENSITY	DURATION

NOTES:

ROLL AWAY THE PAIN

A foam roll can give you an effective massage, and it won't expect a tip. Do these exercises to improve flexibility and increase muscle elasticity, advises Michael Lovegren, MS, of Kinetic Loop training in Greeley, Colorado. For each move, pause at tender spots for 20 seconds.

Injury: Calf Strain

Place a foam roll under one or both of your lower legs and glide up and down the roll. Keep your toes pulled toward you.

Injury: Shinsplints

Balance on both hands with your shins resting on a foam roll. Roll from just below your knees to your ankles.

WEEK 23	WEEK OF / / TO / /	DAY:

STRENGTH TRAINING

EXERCISE	WEIGHT	WARMUP SETS			WORK SETS		
		SET 1 REPS	SET 2 REPS	SET 3 REPS	SET 1 REPS	SET 2 REPS	SET 3 REPS

NOTES:

CARDIO

TYPE	INTENSITY	DURATION

NOTES:

TRAINING TIP

LOCKING OUT JOINTS IS BAD WHEN LIFTING

The phrase "locking out" is misleading. "In power-lifting, you have to lock out in order to receive credit for a lift," says Tom McCullough, CSCS, a strength-and-conditioning coach in Texas. But professionals know how far to stretch their joints.

"What you don't want to do is hyperextend the joint and go beyond the normal anatomic position," he says. When you press beyond your body's natural finish point, the stress of the load transfers from big muscle groups to bones, joints, and ligaments, which aren't prepared to handle it. Serious damage can occur. Observe your body's natural position before starting a lift, McCullough says. Before a leg press, say, stand up straight and see how your knees look when standing tall. Once you reach that spot, don't go beyond it.

You can also combat the risk of hyperextension by incorporating more free weights into your routine: You're at a higher risk of going past the safe point on weight machines.

WEEK 23 | WEEK OF / / TO / / | DAY:

STRENGTH TRAINING

		WARMUP SETS						WORK SETS					
		SET 1		SET 2		SET 3		SET 1		SET 2		SET 3	
EXERCISE	WEIGHT	REPS		REPS		REPS		REPS		REPS		REPS	

NOTES: _____

CARDIO

TYPE	INTENSITY	DURATION

NOTES: _____

Ask the Trainer

What should I eat after I lift?
—Parnel, Barstow, CA

Research shows that a combination of protein and car-bohydrates is best. The ratio depends on your goals. If you're trying to pack on muscle, have a 1:2 ratio of pro-tein to carbs within 10 minutes after you work out. (For example, have some low-fat milk on cereal.) If you're trying to increase lean body mass while losing body fat, go with a 1:1 or 2:1 protein-to-carb ratio, like the EAS Myoplex Shake. And if you're just trying to lose weight, have a preworkout protein shooter, such as a bottle of Amino Vital Pro, then eat a light meal within an hour after your workout.

WEEK 23	WEEK OF / / TO / /	DAY:

STRENGTH TRAINING

EXERCISE	WEIGHT	WARMUP SETS			WORK SETS		
		SET 1 REPS	SET 2 REPS	SET 3 REPS	SET 1 REPS	SET 2 REPS	SET 3 REPS

NOTES:

CARDIO

TYPE	INTENSITY	DURATION

NOTES:

FUELING UP
GO FISH

Fish oils are already linked to better mental performance and a lowered risk of heart disease. Now, omega-3 fatty acids may help relieve neck and back pain, too. University of Pittsburgh scientists gave 1,200 milligrams of fish oil per day to 125 people with neck or back pain; 75 days later, 60 percent of them reported relief. Omega-3s block inflammation and the accompanying pain, says study author Joseph Maroon, MD. Two Nordic Naturals Ultimate Omega capsules contain 1,400 milligrams of fish oil, and they're lemon flavored to help ease fish burp, a side effect of the supplements.

| WEEK 23 | WEEK OF / / TO / / | DAY: |

STRENGTH TRAINING

EXERCISE	WEIGHT	WARMUP SETS						WORK SETS					
		SET 1		SET 2		SET 3		SET 1		SET 2		SET 3	
		REPS		REPS		REPS		REPS		REPS		REPS	

NOTES: _____

CARDIO

TYPE	INTENSITY	DURATION

NOTES: _____

CORE POWER

STICK CRUNCH

This exercise targets both your upper and lower abdominals. Lie on your back with your feet a few inches off the floor and your knees slightly bent. Hold a broomstick in both hands with your arms extended straight out beyond your head. Crunch your torso upward as you draw your knees up so that the stick moves past them. Pause for a second, then return to the starting position. Do 12 repetitions.

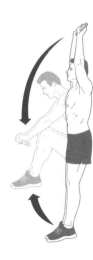

WEEK 24 | WEEK OF / / TO / / | DAY:

STRENGTH TRAINING

EXERCISE	WEIGHT	WARMUP SETS						WORK SETS					
		SET 1		SET 2		SET 3		SET 1		SET 2		SET 3	
		REPS		REPS		REPS		REPS		REPS		REPS	

NOTES:

CARDIO

TYPE	INTENSITY	DURATION

NOTES:

FUELING UP

RACING FUEL

There's more proof that slow-digesting foods provide the best fuel for endurance runners. At England's Loughtorough University, nine men ran for 90 minutes at 70 percent of their VO_2 max, then ate three equal meals and snacks from either a low- or a high-glycemic-index (GI) diet. (Glycemic index is the rate at which carbohydrates convert to blood sugar.) The next morning, the low-GI group ran about 13 minutes longer than the high-GI group did. Researchers say the low-GI group burned more fat and kept more carbohydrate fuel in reserve. A good low-GI meal: beans, cheese, and lettuce on a wheat tortilla.

WEEK 24   WEEK OF / / TO / /   DAY:

STRENGTH TRAINING

EXERCISE	WEIGHT	WARMUP SETS						WORK SETS					
		SET 1		SET 2		SET 3		SET 1		SET 2		SET 3	
		REPS		REPS		REPS		REPS		REPS		REPS	

NOTES: _____

CARDIO

TYPE	INTENSITY	DURATION

NOTES: _____

SCULPT AND STRENGTHEN

BETTER GRIP, BIGGER GAINS

In this workout, you'll hold a barbell in one hand like a dumbbell. For each exercise, do three sets of six reps with each arm. Rest for 60 seconds between sets and for at least a day between workouts.

SUITCASE DEADLIFT

Grasp a barbell with your right hand at your side. Move your hips back and bend your knees until your thighs are parallel to the floor. Pause for a second. Then, without rounding your back, drive your feet into the floor and stand.

UNILATERAL SHOULDER PRESS

Stand holding a barbell with your right hand next to your face and the bar perpendicular to your shoulders. Press the bar up until your arm is straight, then lower it to the starting position.

SINGLE-ARM BARBELL ROW

Holding a barbell with your right hand, place your left knee and left hand on a bench. Keeping your back straight, balance the bar as you pull your elbow up past your torso. Hold for a second, then lower.

WEEK 24 WEEK OF / / TO / / DAY:

STRENGTH TRAINING

EXERCISE	WEIGHT	WARMUP SETS			WORK SETS		
		SET 1 REPS	SET 2 REPS	SET 3 REPS	SET 1 REPS	SET 2 REPS	SET 3 REPS

NOTES:

CARDIO

TYPE	INTENSITY	DURATION

NOTES:

TRAINING TIP
KEEP THE BEAT

Your heart rate is a reliable gauge of workout intensity and fitness. So measure it correctly—with a heart-rate monitor. Taking your pulse with your fingers after exercise greatly underestimates your heart rate, according to the *Scandinavian Journal of Medicine and Science in Sports*. Study subjects who took their pulses at the wrist and neck 15 seconds after treadmill runs underestimated rates by 27 beats per minute (bpm) for low-intensity runs and by 20 bpm at higher intensities. Their hearts slowed quickly after the run, says study author Hirofumi Tanaka, PhD. Instead, use a monitor like Polar's new F11 ($180, www.polarusa.com). It has a comfy chest strap and won't pick up interference from other monitors.

WEEK 24 | WEEK OF / / TO / / | DAY:

STRENGTH TRAINING

EXERCISE	WEIGHT	WARMUP SETS			WORK SETS		
		SET 1	SET 2	SET 3	SET 1	SET 2	SET 3
		REPS	REPS	REPS	REPS	REPS	REPS

NOTES: _____

CARDIO

TYPE	INTENSITY	DURATION

NOTES: _____

WEEK 25		WEEK OF / / TO / /		DAY:	

STRENGTH TRAINING

EXERCISE	WEIGHT	WARMUP SETS			WORK SETS		
		SET 1 REPS	SET 2 REPS	SET 3 REPS	SET 1 REPS	SET 2 REPS	SET 3 REPS

NOTES: _____

CARDIO

TYPE	INTENSITY	DURATION

NOTES: _____

IS YOUR DIET WORKING?

Here are two signs that you need to rethink what you have—or haven't—been chewing on.

HAIR EVERYWHERE—EXCEPT ON TOP

The likely culprit: A low-calorie regimen. "Dipping below 1,000 calories a day deprives your body of the energy and nutrients it needs to regenerate your hair cells," says Cindy Moore, RD, director of nutrition therapy at the Cleveland Clinic Foundation, in Ohio.
The fix: Never drop below 1,800 calories a day.

YOU CAN'T CONCENTRATE

The likely culprit: Skipping breakfast. Researchers at the University of Bristol in the United Kingdom found that people who skipped breakfast had focus problems and fumbled tasks later in the day. "After a long night of not eating, you need to give your brain glucose, or food sugar, to function," says Moore.
The fix: Eat within an hour of waking. Rushed? Make it easy: a handful of almonds and an apple.

SCULPT AND STRENGTHEN

SHORE UP YOUR ROTATOR CUFF

FOUR-WAY PICKUP AND REACH

Stand with your left heel 2 feet in front of your right toes, knees bent, and hold a 5-pound dumbbell in your right hand just outside of your left calf. Lift across your body—rotating your wrist so your thumb points behind you—until your arm is extended over your right shoulder. Reverse to the starting position. Repeat with the dumbbell still in your right hand but your right leg in front. That's one rep. Then do the series holding the weight in your left hand. Do two sets of 12 reps.

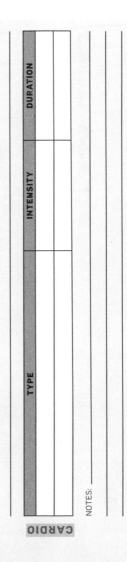

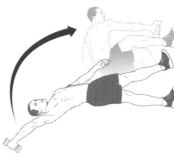

WEEK 25 | WEEK OF / / TO / / | DAY:

STRENGTH TRAINING

EXERCISE	WEIGHT	WARMUP SETS			WORK SETS		
		SET 1 REPS	SET 2 REPS	SET 3 REPS	SET 1 REPS	SET 2 REPS	SET 3 REPS

NOTES: _____

CARDIO

TYPE	INTENSITY	DURATION

NOTES: _____

BODY MOVING

GET FITTER, FASTER

We took two of the best sports for burning fat and asked experts for tweaks that produce major results. Here's the payoff for a fit, 170-pound man.

RUNNING. Run ladders. "Ladders create sustained intensity," says Mindy Solkin, owner and head coach of www.therunningcenter.com. Use the first and last miles of a 4-mile run to warm up and cool down. In between, run 30 seconds fast, 30 seconds slow, 45 seconds fast and slow, and then 60 seconds of both. Follow with 1 or 2 minutes at recovery pace before reversing the ladder (60, 60, 45, 45, 30, 30). Ladders boost your burn by 60 percent. That's 432 calories per half hour, compared with 270 calories while jogging.

SWIMMING. Swim with fins. Fins create more resistance, requiring you to use more muscle mass and energy when moving through the water, says Doug Stern, a swim instructor in New York City. "You need to train your muscles to move continuously," Stern says. "Fins tap into the muscle and energy in the legs that are often ignored by amateur swimmers." You'll burn 25 percent more calories. That's 388 calories in 30 minutes, compared with 310 calories without fins.

WEEK 25 WEEK OF / / TO / /   DAY:

STRENGTH TRAINING

EXERCISE	WEIGHT	WARMUP SETS			WORK SETS		
		SET 1 REPS	SET 2 REPS	SET 3 REPS	SET 1 REPS	SET 2 REPS	SET 3 REPS

NOTES:

CARDIO

TYPE	INTENSITY	DURATION

NOTES:

FUELING UP

DOUBLE YOUR RESULTS—INSTANTLY

Watch the clock before and after your workout, and your arms will grow bigger. In a new study, 17 men drank two protein shakes a day—either immediately before and after their workouts, or at least 5 hours outside of their training sessions. After 10 weeks, the researchers noticed a stark contrast: Men who sandwich their workouts with protein build nearly twice as much muscle as those who don't. "Your body uses nutrients to build muscle most effectively in the hour on either side of your workout," says Alan Hayes, PhD. So fuel up to look great.

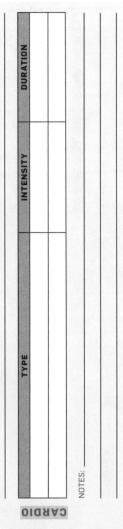

WEEK 25 | WEEK OF / / TO / / | DAY:

STRENGTH TRAINING

EXERCISE	WEIGHT	WARMUP SETS			WORK SETS		
		SET 1 REPS	SET 2 REPS	SET 3 REPS	SET 1 REPS	SET 2 REPS	SET 3 REPS

NOTES: _____

CARDIO

TYPE	INTENSITY	DURATION

NOTES: _____

TRAINING TIP

LIFT FIRST, RUN SECOND

We've long touted the fat-loss benefits of weight training. But now Japanese scientists have discovered that lifting weights before you run helps you burn more flab while you pound the pavement. In fact, men who performed a weight-lifting routine and then hopped on a stationary bike burned twice as much fat as those who only pedaled. Resistance exercise stimulates the release of fat-burning hormones, which trigger your body to use more lard for energy.

WEEK 26 | WEEK OF / / TO / / | DAY:

STRENGTH TRAINING

EXERCISE	WEIGHT	WARMUP SETS			WORK SETS		
		SET 1 REPS	SET 2 REPS	SET 3 REPS	SET 1 REPS	SET 2 REPS	SET 3 REPS

NOTES: _____

CARDIO

TYPE	INTENSITY	DURATION

NOTES: _____

Ask the Trainer

The grip attachments at the row machine—which do I use?

—Bruce, Boston, MA

Depends on what you want. But before you worry about grips, master the fundamentals of the seated row. Sit upright with your knees bent, pushing your chest out and pulling your shoulders back while maintaining an upright torso throughout the move. "Rounding your lower back at any time during the exercise can cause injury," says Craig Ballantyne, CSCS, owner of www.turbulencetraining.com. The seated row trains your back (lats, rhomboids, and traps) ard shoulders (deltoids), providing greater spine support. By changing the angle of your arms, these grip options target different areas of your back and shoulders.

WEEK 26 | **WEEK OF / / TO / /** | **DAY:**

STRENGTH TRAINING

EXERCISE	WEIGHT	WARMUP SETS			WORK SETS		
		SET 1 REPS	SET 2 REPS	SET 3 REPS	SET 1 REPS	SET 2 REPS	SET 3 REPS

NOTES:

CARDIO

TYPE	INTENSITY	DURATION

NOTES:

FUELING UP

NUTS

Superpowers: boosts testosterone, builds muscle, burns fat

Secret weapons: protein, monounsaturated fat, vitamin E, niacin, magnesium

Fights against: obesity, muscle loss, wrinkles, cardiovascular disease

Sidekicks: cashew and almond butters

HOW TO USE THEM

- CREATE A SAUCE. Sure, there's nothing wrong with PB&J. But try eating peanut butter in ways you might not have thought of before. Like this: Microwave 2 tablespoons of peanut butter until soft, then mix well with ¼ cup low-sodium soy sauce and some crushed red pepper flakes. Toss with whole-wheat noodles or use it as a dip for precooked chicken strips.
- EAT IT AU NATUREL. In a rush? Just pop a spoonful or two.

| WEEK 26 | WEEK OF / / TO / / | DAY: |

STRENGTH TRAINING

EXERCISE	WEIGHT	WARMUP SETS			WORK SETS		
		SET 1 REPS	SET 2 REPS	SET 3 REPS	SET 1 REPS	SET 2 REPS	SET 3 REPS

NOTES:

CARDIO

TYPE	INTENSITY	DURATION

NOTES:

TRAINING TIP

THE SCIENCE OF SQUAT

Keep your head up: Looking down when you squat puts you at greater risk of injury, report researchers at Miami University of Ohio. In a recent study, scientists discovered that gazing downward while squatting—compared with looking straight ahead or up—causes you to lean forward 4 to 5 degrees. This increases the strain on your lower back and limits the amount of weight you can use. "Focus on a point straight ahead and maintain that focus as you lower your body into the squat," says study author Darryn Fiske, CSCS, MS. Once you reach the bottom position, tilt your head back toward the bar, then drive your hips forward to push yourself back up.

WEEK 26	WEEK OF / / TO / /	DAY:

STRENGTH TRAINING

| | | WARMUP SETS | | | WORK SETS | | |
EXERCISE	WEIGHT	SET 1 REPS	SET 2 REPS	SET 3 REPS	SET 1 REPS	SET 2 REPS	SET 3 REPS

NOTES:

CARDIO

TYPE	INTENSITY	DURATION

NOTES:

SHOE SURGERY

If you have a hard time bending your forefoot, consider surgery—on your shoe. Cutting the sole of your running shoe can lower your injury risk, according to the journal *The Physician and Sports Medicine*. Slicing the sole horizontally at the ball of the foot provides greater flexibility, says study author Russell Nelson, PT, PhD. Achilles tendinitis and plantar fasciitis can be caused by a rigid sole that prevents the foot from extending fully and strains the foot and calf. Or buy Nike's new Free model, which offers the best in forefoot flexibility, he says.

WEEK 27   WEEK OF / / TO / /   DAY:

STRENGTH TRAINING

EXERCISE	WEIGHT	WARMUP SETS						WORK SETS					
		SET 1		SET 2		SET 3		SET 1		SET 2		SET 3	
		REPS		REPS		REPS		REPS		REPS		REPS	

NOTES:

CARDIO

TYPE	INTENSITY	DURATION

NOTES:

FUELING UP
LEAN CUISINE

Reserve a table for two: Dinner dates can make you thin. In a recent study, researchers at the State University of New York at Buffalo observed that men downed 35 percent fewer calories when eating with their significant others, compared with eating with their buddies. "People tend to match their own intake to the amount their dining partners eat," says study author Sarah-Jeanne Salvy, PhD. "Women may be more cognizant of how gluttonous they appear to their partners." One way to avoid pigging out on guys' night: Choose an entrée for yourself and skip communal foods like nachos, wings, and pizza, which encourage you to take eating cues from your porcine pals.

WEEK 27 | WEEK OF / / TO / / | DAY:

STRENGTH TRAINING

EXERCISE	WEIGHT	WARMUP SETS			WORK SETS		
		SET 1 REPS	SET 2 REPS	SET 3 REPS	SET 1 REPS	SET 2 REPS	SET 3 REPS

NOTES:

CARDIO

TYPE	INTENSITY	DURATION

NOTES:

Ask the Trainer

How can I throw farther?
—*Gene, Brooklyn, NY*

Try the cable wood chop in explosive fashion. Training your body to rotate more explosively through your core can add distance and velocity to your throw. You'll also protect your shoulder from injury, says Mike Gough, CSCS. Attach a rope handle to a high-pulley cable. Stand with your left side toward the stack and your feet slightly more than shoulder-width apart. Grab the rope with both hands. Keeping your arms straight and your abs tight, bend your knees as you forcefully pull the handle down and across your body toward your right lower leg. Reverse the motion and finish your reps before switching sides. Do two or three sets of five to seven repetitions.

WEEK 27 WEEK OF / / TO / / DAY:

STRENGTH TRAINING

EXERCISE	WEIGHT	WARM-UP SETS			WORK SETS		
		SET 1	SET 2	SET 3	SET 1	SET 2	SET 3
		REPS	REPS	REPS	REPS	REPS	REPS

NOTES:

CARDIO

TYPE	INTENSITY	DURATION

NOTES:

A SECOND WIND

Do you think lifting in the morning wipes you out for an afternoon run? Turns out the exact opposite may be true.

Dave Pearson, CSCS, PhD, director of the strength-research laboratory at Ball State University in Muncie, Indiana, found that if you lift in the morning and run in the afternoon, your muscles will have a greater fuel reserve—nearly twice as much in his study—than if you reverse this order, running first.

Dr. Pearson studied men who did a morning weight session, recovered for about 6 hours while feasting on carbs, and then ran and biked later in the day. A portion of the lactate they produced while lifting was later converted into glycogen—the fuel that drives muscles and can propel you through a cardio session. His conclusion: If you lift until your tank's empty in the a.m., it will fill itself up in time for your p.m. session.

WEEK 27 | **WEEK OF** / / **TO** / / | **DAY:** [   ]

STRENGTH TRAINING

EXERCISE	WEIGHT	WARMUP SETS			WORK SETS		
		SET 1 REPS	SET 2 REPS	SET 3 REPS	SET 1 REPS	SET 2 REPS	SET 3 REPS

NOTES: _____

CARDIO

TYPE	INTENSITY	DURATION

NOTES: _____

WEEK 28 | WEEK OF / / TO / / | DAY:

SPOTLIGHT EXERCISE

DUMBBELL UNDERHAND PUSHUP

Grab a dumbbell in each hand and get in pushup position with your palms facing forward. The dumbbells should align with the middle of your sternum, and your arms should be spaced about shoulder-width apart.

Without allowing your elbows to flare to the sides, lower your chest to the floor. (Your hands should touch the sides of your chest at the bottom of the movement.) Then push yourself back up.

STRENGTH TRAINING

EXERCISE	WEIGHT	WARMUP SETS			WORK SETS		
		SET 1 REPS	SET 2 REPS	SET 3 REPS	SET 1 REPS	SET 2 REPS	SET 3 REPS

NOTES:

CARDIO

TYPE	INTENSITY	DURATION

NOTES:

TRAINING TIP

FIRE UP YOUR MUSCLES

Calisthenics are a better warmup than traditional stretching, report researchers at the United States Military Academy. When scientists examined different methods of preparing for exercise, they found that first performing calisthenics—also known as dynamic stretching—helped men sprint faster, jump higher, and throw harder. However, a static-stretching warmup—the stretch-and-hold variety—provided no such benefit. The likely explanation: Dynamic stretching enhances nervous-system activity, which allows you to recruit more muscle fibers, says study author Danny McMillian PT, DSc, OCS. So before you hit the weights, field, or court, do 30 seconds each of jumping jacks, arm circles, pushups, lunges, and body-weight squats.

WEEK 28 | WEEK OF / / TO / / | DAY:

STRENGTH TRAINING

EXERCISE	WEIGHT	WARMUP SETS			WORK SETS		
		SET 1 REPS	SET 2 REPS	SET 3 REPS	SET 1 REPS	SET 2 REPS	SET 3 REPS

NOTES:

CARDIO

TYPE	INTENSITY	DURATION

NOTES:

WAIT FOR RESULTS

Be patient. According to a new study by researchers at Arkansas State University, the oft-recommended 48 hours of rest between workouts may not be enough. After doing three to six sets of leg presses, 67 percent of the men studied needed 96 hours for their leg strength to fully recover. "The next question that needs to be addressed is, 'Do you have to be completely recovered to lift again and see gains?'" says Brian Church, PhD, the study's lead author. Until researchers know for sure, Church suggests keeping a log of your total volume (sets × reps × weight lifted). If volume dips, take some time off to thoroughly recoup your strength.

WEEK 28 | WEEK OF / / TO / / | DAY:

STRENGTH TRAINING

EXERCISE	WEIGHT	WARMUP SETS			WORK SETS		
		SET 1 REPS	SET 2 REPS	SET 3 REPS	SET 1 REPS	SET 2 REPS	SET 3 REPS

NOTES: _____

CARDIO

TYPE	INTENSITY	DURATION

NOTES: _____

FUELING UP
CHAMPION OF BREAKFAST

Yolking your diet could rein in your appetite. Saint Louis University scientists found that people who eat eggs as part of their breakfast consume fewer calories the rest of the day than those who skip the eggs. In the study, people were given one of two breakfasts: (1) two scrambled eggs, two slices of toast, and a tablespoon of reduced-calorie fruit spread; or (2) a bagel, 2 tablespoons of cream cheese, and 3 ounces of nonfat yogurt. Even though the breakfasts were equal in calories, the egg eaters consumed 264 fewer calories by the end of the day. The researchers aren't sure why eating eggs appears to reduce hunger and food intake, but they think that the meal's higher protein and fat content may lead to greater satiety.

WEEK 28 | WEEK OF / / TO / / | DAY:

STRENGTH TRAINING

EXERCISE	WEIGHT	WARMUP SETS			WORK SETS		
		SET 1 REPS	SET 2 REPS	SET 3 REPS	SET 1 REPS	SET 2 REPS	SET 3 REPS

NOTES: _____

CARDIO

TYPE	INTENSITY	DURATION

NOTES: _____

Ask the Trainer

I know you're not supposed to eat before going to bed, but I have to work out at 11:00 p.m. What can I eat after my workout?

—Filip, New Orleans, LA

Just make sure you eat your last complete meal of the day an hour or two before your workout. A small post-workout, presnooze snack is fine. Try a cup of low-fat yogurt and a banana, or some cereal and an orange, or a protein shake. Then shower up and hit the sheets.

WEEK 29	WEEK OF / / TO / /	DAY:

STRENGTH TRAINING

EXERCISE	WEIGHT	WARM-UP SETS			WORK SETS		
		SET 1 REPS	SET 2 REPS	SET 3 REPS	SET 1 REPS	SET 2 REPS	SET 3 REPS

NOTES: _____

CARDIO

TYPE	INTENSITY	DURATION

NOTES: _____

SPOTLIGHT EXERCISE

WINNING ROTATION

Bend your elbow at a right angle so your upper arm is parallel to the floor, like you're giving a high five. Rotate your hand forward and down. If you fall short of 180 degrees of rotation, your rotator-cuff muscles are tight. Do the stretch below twice a day.

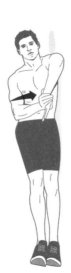

Lie on your side with your upper arm on the floor and your elbow bent 90 degrees, fingers pointing up. Gently push your hand toward the floor until you feel a stretch in your rear shoulder. Hold for 30 seconds.

WEEK 29 | WEEK OF / / TO / / DAY: [ ]

STRENGTH TRAINING

EXERCISE	WEIGHT	WARMUP SETS			WORK SETS		
		SET 1 REPS	SET 2 REPS	SET 3 REPS	SET 1 REPS	SET 2 REPS	SET 3 REPS

NOTES:

CARDIO

TYPE	INTENSITY	DURATION

NOTES:

Ask the Trainer

Is there any calorie-burn difference in working out in the heat versus with the AC on?
— *Bryan, Las Vegas, NV*

Yes, but it's negligible. If the workouts are identical, performing in the heat will boost your heart rate and have you breathing heavier than you would in cooler locales. The upside of this extra exertion: You'll burn more calories. The downside: Hot weather can also wear you out faster, cutting your workout short. "If a cool environment permits you to work out at a higher intensity or for a longer duration, then overall caloric burn would be greater in that environment," says Thayne Munce, PhD, clinical assistant professor in the department of movement sciences at the University of Illinois at Chicago. The difference between hot- and cold-weather calorie burn is thought to be slim, but if you want to eke all the weight-loss benefit you can out of your exercise, acclimate yourself to the heat by slowly increasing the intensity of your outdoor workouts. Build up your routine over 14 days to maximize your acclimation.

WEEK 29 WEEK OF / / TO / /   DAY:

STRENGTH TRAINING

EXERCISE	WEIGHT	WARMUP SETS SET 1 REPS	SET 2 REPS	SET 3 REPS	WORK SETS SET 1 REPS	SET 2 REPS	SET 3 REPS

NOTES:

CARDIO

TYPE	INTENSITY	DURATION

NOTES:

FUELING UP
EXTRA-PROTEIN (WHEY) POWDER

Superpowers: builds muscle, burns fat

Secret weapons: protein, cysteine, glutathione

Fights against: obesity

Sidekick: ricotta cheese (part skim)

HOW TO USE IT

- Mix it up. Add some to your smoothies. Every day.
- Stir it up. Blend a teaspoonful into a cup of pudding or yogurt.
- Hide some in your oatmeal—mix a spoonful with the dry ingredients, then cook.

Tirami-Smoothie

¾ cup part-skim ricotta cheese
2 tablespoons reduced-fat yogurt
1 tablespoon slivered unsalted almonds
2 teaspoons chocolate whey-protein powder
2 teaspoons ground flaxseed
½ teaspoon finely ground coffee beans
6 ice cubes

Chuck everything into a blender. Mix well.

WEEK 29	WEEK OF / / TO / /	DAY:

STRENGTH TRAINING

EXERCISE	WEIGHT	WARMUP SETS			WORK SETS		
		SET 1 REPS	SET 2 REPS	SET 3 REPS	SET 1 REPS	SET 2 REPS	SET 3 REPS

NOTES: _____

CARDIO

TYPE	INTENSITY	DURATION

NOTES: _____

PERSISTENCE PAYS

Exercise works as a weight-loss strategy—if you actually do it. A study by the Centers for Disease Control and Prevention found that only 19 percent of people exercising to lose weight do the recommended 60 minutes a day. And only 57 percent work out for more than 150 minutes a week. "People trying to lose weight often become discouraged when their progress is slow," the study authors write. They suggest breaking up exercise into short sessions of 8 to 10 minutes.

WEEK 30	WEEK OF / / TO / /	DAY:

STRENGTH TRAINING

EXERCISE	WEIGHT	WARMUP SETS						WORK SETS					
		SET 1		SET 2		SET 3		SET 1		SET 2		SET 3	
		REPS		REPS		REPS		REPS		REPS		REPS	

NOTES:

CARDIO

TYPE	INTENSITY	DURATION

NOTES:

FUELING UP
FLUSH THAT SOY SHAKE

Researchers compared how soy protein and casein protein (from dairy products) are converted into a waste product called urea. The study found that soy protein is converted far more readily into urea and eliminated during protein synthesis (how protein is turned into muscle). The article, in *Human Nutrition and Metabolism*, also says that protein synthesis is more than three times greater with casein protein than with soy.

WEEK 30	WEEK OF / / TO / /	DAY:

STRENGTH TRAINING

EXERCISE	WEIGHT	WARMUP SETS			WORK SETS		
		SET 1 REPS	SET 2 REPS	SET 3 REPS	SET 1 REPS	SET 2 REPS	SET 3 REPS

NOTES: _____

CARDIO

TYPE	INTENSITY	DURATION

NOTES: _____

Ask the Trainer

Caffeine is in diet supplements, so why do some diets forbid coffee?
—Eric, Raleigh, NC

Caffeine stimulates the central nervous system, increasing your basal metabolic rate so you burn more calories. (Exercise is better at this, without the negative side effects of weight-loss supplements.) Some diet authors claim that excess caffeine can cause a drop in blood-sugar levels, leaving you craving sweets, but this has not been substantiated. If you're eating a well-balanced meal along with your caffeine, you shouldn't have a problem. Plus, chlorogenic acid, an antioxidant compound found in coffee, may improve glucose metabolism to further aid in keeping the pounds off.

WEEK 30

WEEK OF / / **TO** / /   **DAY:**

STRENGTH TRAINING

EXERCISE	WEIGHT	WARMUP SETS						WORK SETS					
		SET 1		SET 2		SET 3		SET 1		SET 2		SET 3	
		REPS		REPS		REPS		REPS		REPS		REPS	

NOTES:

CARDIO

TYPE	INTENSITY	DURATION

NOTES:

CORE POWER

TWO-FOR-ONE ABS EXERCISE

WEIGHTED ONE-SIDED CRUNCH

This exercise targets both the upper abs and the obliques. Lie with your knees bent and your feet flat on the floor, and hold a dumbbell with both hands by your right shoulder. Curl your torso up and rotate to the left. Lower yourself, finish the set on that side, then switch directions and repeat, holding the dumbbell by your left shoulder. Perform three sets of eight repetitions to each side.

WEEK 30 | WEEK OF / / TO / / | DAY:

STRENGTH TRAINING

EXERCISE	WEIGHT	WARMUP SETS			WORK SETS		
		SET 1 REPS	SET 2 REPS	SET 3 REPS	SET 1 REPS	SET 2 REPS	SET 3 REPS

NOTES:

CARDIO

TYPE	INTENSITY	DURATION

NOTES:

SCULPT AND STRENGTHEN

POWER POINTERS

Pay closer attention to your exercise technique and you may notice something: Men who review proper lifting form before bench-pressing may increase barbell velocity by 183 percent, report researchers at Barry University in Miami Shores, Florida. "Faster bar speed helps you overcome inertia and blast through sticking points," says strength coach Jason Ferruggia. The next time you bench-press, recall three form cues: Pull your shoulder blades down and together, keep your elbows close to your sides as you lower the weight, and try to rip the bar apart as you push it straight up.

WEEK 31 | WEEK OF / / TO / / | DAY:

STRENGTH TRAINING

EXERCISE	WEIGHT	WARMUP SETS						WORK SETS					
		SET 1	REPS	SET 2	REPS	SET 3	REPS	SET 1	REPS	SET 2	REPS	SET 3	REPS

NOTES:

CARDIO

TYPE	INTENSITY	DURATION

NOTES:

FUELING UP
A NUTTY PREWORKOUT SNACK

High in cholesterol-scouring fiber and muscle-building protein, peanuts are the ideal snack during midafternoon doldrums. But what if they're roasted, salted, or candy-coated?

EAT THESE

Oil-roasted, with salt (1 oz): 170 calories, 8 g protein, 4 g carbs, 15 g total fat, 2 g saturated fat, 3 g fiber, 91 mg sodium

Butter toffee–coated (1 oz): 140 calories, 4 g protein, 16 g carbs, 7 g total fat, 1 g saturated fat, 2 g fiber, 20 mg sodium

Goobers (1.375-oz packet): 200 calories, 5 g protein, 19 g carbs, 13 g total fat, 5 g saturated fat, 2 g fiber, 16 mg sodium

NOT THESE

Dry-roasted, with salt (1 oz): 166 calories, 7 g protein, 6 g carbs, 14 g total fat, 2 g saturated fat, 2 g fiber, 230 mg sodium

Yogurt-coated (1 oz): 154 calories, 4 g protein, 12 g carbs, 10 g total fat, 5 g saturated fat, 1 g fiber, 16 mg sodium

Peanut M&Ms (1.67-oz packet): 243 calories, 4 g protein, 28 g carbs, 12 g total fat, 5 g saturated fat, 2 g fiber, 23 mg sodium

---

WEEK 31 | **WEEK OF** / / **TO** / / | **DAY:**

STRENGTH TRAINING

EXERCISE	WEIGHT	WARMUP SETS			WORK SETS		
		SET 1 REPS	SET 2 REPS	SET 3 REPS	SET 1 REPS	SET 2 REPS	SET 3 REPS

NOTES:

CARDIO

TYPE	INTENSITY	DURATION

NOTES:

CORE POWER

KNEELING CABLE CRUNCH

Kneel facing the pulley and hold the ends of a rope attached to the high cable along the sides of your face. Bend forward, aiming your chest at your pelvis. Return to the starting position, then repeat the movement, this time aiming your chest toward your left knee. Return, then repeat to your right. That's one repetition. Perform three sets of eight repetitions.

WEEK 31 | **WEEK OF / / TO / /** | **DAY:**

STRENGTH TRAINING

EXERCISE	WEIGHT	WARMUP SETS			WORK SETS		
		SET 1 REPS	SET 2 REPS	SET 3 REPS	SET 1 REPS	SET 2 REPS	SET 3 REPS

NOTES:

CARDIO

TYPE	INTENSITY	DURATION

NOTES:

RETURN TO SLENDER

When scientists at McMaster University in Hamilton, Ontario, assessed the food intakes of 617 people, they found that eating more protein may reduce the fat around your midsection. People who ate 20 grams more protein every day than the group average had 6 percent lower waist-to-hip ratios. Most made small adjustments, such as replacing ¾ cup of rice with half a chicken breast, says Anwar Merchant, PhD.

WEEK 31	WEEK OF / / TO / /	DAY:

STRENGTH TRAINING

EXERCISE	WEIGHT	WARMUP SETS			WORK SETS		
		SET 1 REPS	SET 2 REPS	SET 3 REPS	SET 1 REPS	SET 2 REPS	SET 3 REPS

NOTES: _____

CARDIO

TYPE	INTENSITY	DURATION

NOTES: _____

FUELING UP

PEEL AWAY THE FAT

Make that two apples a day. UCLA researchers discovered that small differences in fruit and fiber intake can dictate whether people are overweight. In the study, normal-weight people reported eating, on average, two servings of fruit and 12 grams of fiber a day; those who were overweight had just one serving and 9 grams. Credit that extra 3 grams of fiber—the amount in one apple or orange—as the difference maker. Fiber slows digestion and enhances satiety, says study author Beth Gillham, PhD, RD.

WEEK 32 | WEEK OF / / TO / / | DAY:

STRENGTH TRAINING

EXERCISE	WEIGHT	WARMUP SETS						WORK SETS					
		SET 1		SET 2		SET 3		SET 1		SET 2		SET 3	
		REPS		REPS		REPS		REPS		REPS		REPS	

NOTES:

CARDIO

TYPE	INTENSITY	DURATION

NOTES:

THE ABS VITAMIN

Fat-loss supplements may soon feature a new ingredient. People who take 500 milligrams of vitamin C daily burn 39 percent more fat during exercise than those who ingest only small amounts of the nutrient, according to a recent study by Arizona State University. "Low levels of vitamin C may impede your body's ability to use fat as energy," says author Carol Johnston, PhD. And chances are, most men could use more C. That's because the average guy consumes 102 milligrams of the vitamin daily, and his top source—orange juice—contains just 82 milligrams per 8-ounce serving. Worse, previous research shows that OJ loses up to 50 percent of its vitamin C content during processing and handling, and 2 percent more every day afterward. The best way to boost your intake? Try a supplement such as Buffered C-500, available at www.iherb.com ($6 for 100 500-milligram capsules).

WEEK 32 | WEEK OF / / TO / / | DAY:

STRENGTH TRAINING

EXERCISE	WEIGHT	WARMUP SETS			WORK SETS		
		SET 1 REPS	SET 2 REPS	SET 3 REPS	SET 1 REPS	SET 2 REPS	SET 3 REPS

NOTES: _____

CARDIO

TYPE	INTENSITY	DURATION

NOTES: _____

GO FOR A STROLLER

Some serious runners balk at jogging strollers. But a new study in the *Journal of Sports Medicine and Physical Fitness* found that running while pushing a stroller burns more calories and doesn't hurt your running form. Researchers had 10 athletes run with and without a stroller for 30 minutes. The added resistance of the stroller boosted both their heart rates and lactate concentrations without affecting stride length. "Physiologically, no negatives come from pushing a stroller," says study author John Smith, PhD, who recommends a one-armed grip. "The opposite arm is then free to swing, helping to counterbalance your legs."

WEEK 32 | WEEK OF / / TO / / | DAY:

STRENGTH TRAINING

EXERCISE	WEIGHT	WARMUP SETS			WORK SETS		
		SET 1 REPS	SET 2 REPS	SET 3 REPS	SET 1 REPS	SET 2 REPS	SET 3 REPS

NOTES: _____

CARDIO

TYPE	INTENSITY	DURATION

NOTES: _____

TRAINING TIP

TELL YOURSELF OFF

So you missed a workout and now you want to exorcise your guilt. Step 1: Remember that muscle needs to rest in order to rebuild and grow. Step 2: Know that "it would take a 10- to 15-day hiatus from working out for you to see any significant effects on your body," says John Silva, PhD, professor of sports psychology at the University of North Carolina at Chapel Hill. Step 3: Tell yourself that even God took a day off from bench-pressing mountain ranges.

| WEEK 32 | WEEK OF / / TO / / | DAY: |

STRENGTH TRAINING

EXERCISE	WEIGHT	WARM-UP SETS			WORK SETS		
		SET 1 REPS	SET 2 REPS	SET 3 REPS	SET 1 REPS	SET 2 REPS	SET 3 REPS

NOTES:

CARDIO

TYPE	INTENSITY	DURATION

NOTES:

Ask the Trainer

What's a good exercise to improve my golf swing?
—Richie, Mechanicsburg, PA

Try the twister. "The golf swing is all about rotation," says Houston-based personal trainer Carter Hays, CSCS. "A golfer has to rotate virtually every joint to its functional capacity if he wants to come close to his potential." This exercise will help you rotate with more strength and through a greater range of motion at the hips and shoulders. Focus on initiating the move from your hips while keeping the rest of your body stable. Perform three sets of 12 repetitions, 3 days a week.

TWISTER

Get into a modified pushup position with your shins on a Swiss ball and your hands on the floor, directly beneath your shoulders. Slide your legs about halfway down the sides of the ball. Keeping your legs straight and your navel pulled in toward your spine, move the ball to the left by attempting to touch your left foot to the floor. Next, try to touch your right foot to the floor so the ball moves to the right, and return to the starting position. That's one repetition.

WEEK 33 | WEEK OF / / TO / / | DAY:

STRENGTH TRAINING

EXERCISE	WEIGHT	WARMUP SETS						WORK SETS					
		SET 1		SET 2		SET 3		SET 1		SET 2		SET 3	
		REPS		REPS		REPS		REPS		REPS		REPS	

NOTES:

CARDIO

TYPE	INTENSITY	DURATION

NOTES:

FUELING UP
SCALE DOWN

Here's another fish-oil endorsement: Omega-3 fatty acids may help you lose weight. A Czech study revealed that omega-3s may help stymie the body's natural tendency to store fat. Increasing omega-3 intake in mice from 1 to 12 percent of total fat consumption appeared to deprogram fat-hoarding genes. Next up for researchers: determining whether the effect can be replicated in humans.

WEEK 33 | WEEK OF / / TO / / | DAY:

STRENGTH TRAINING

EXERCISE	WEIGHT	WARMUP SETS			WORK SETS		
		SET 1 REPS	SET 2 REPS	SET 3 REPS	SET 1 REPS	SET 2 REPS	SET 3 REPS

NOTES:

CARDIO

TYPE	INTENSITY	DURATION

NOTES:

Ask the Trainer

I'd like to start lifting, but my schedule only frees up after 9:00 p.m. Is it okay to work out this late at night?
—*Clyde, Raleigh, NC*

If 9:00 p.m. is your only time, then it's the best time. You may feel slightly more energized for a couple of hours after you work out, but you also might get a deeper night's sleep than usual. If you're too alert, try to tweak your day so you can work out just before you need the most energy.

WEEK 33	WEEK OF / / TO / /	DAY:

STRENGTH TRAINING

EXERCISE	WEIGHT	WARMUP SETS						WORK SETS					
		SET 1		SET 2		SET 3		SET 1		SET 2		SET 3	
		REPS		REPS		REPS		REPS		REPS		REPS	

NOTES:

CARDIO

TYPE	INTENSITY	DURATION

NOTES:

SPOTLIGHT EXERCISE

RAISED KNEE-IN

This exercise works your lower abs. Lie on your back with your arms close to your sides, and your palms down just under your lower back and butt. Press the small of your back against the floor and extend your legs outward, with your heels about 3 inches above the floor. Keeping your lower back against the floor, lift your left knee toward your chest. Your right leg should remain hovering above the floor. Hold, then straighten your left leg to the starting position and repeat with your right leg. Keep your abs tight throughout the exercise. Do 15 to 20 repetitions with each leg.

WEEK 33 | WEEK OF / / TO / / | DAY:

STRENGTH TRAINING

EXERCISE	WEIGHT	WARMUP SETS						WORK SETS					
		SET 1		SET 2		SET 3		SET 1		SET 2		SET 3	
		REPS		REPS		REPS		REPS		REPS		REPS	

NOTES:

CARDIO

TYPE	INTENSITY	DURATION

NOTES:

CORE POWER

A HARDER CORE CHALLENGE

Master the side bridge to build better abs.

KNEELING SIDE BRIDGE

Lie on your side with your forearm on the floor and elbow under your shoulder, knees bent 90 degrees. Contract your glutes and keep your abs stiff throughout. Raise your hips until your torso is straight from shoulders to knees.

SIDE BRIDGE

Lie on your side with your forearm on the floor under your shoulder, and your feet stacked together. Contract your glutes and abs and push your hip off the floor, creating a straight line from ankle to shoulder and keeping your head in line with your spine.

ELEVATED SIDE BRIDGE

Do the side bridge, but stack your feet on a bench.

WEEK 34 | WEEK OF / / TO / / | DAY:

STRENGTH TRAINING

EXERCISE	WEIGHT	WARMUP SETS			WORK SETS		
		SET 1 REPS	SET 2 REPS	SET 3 REPS	SET 1 REPS	SET 2 REPS	SET 3 REPS

NOTES:

CARDIO

TYPE	INTENSITY	DURATION

NOTES:

Ask the Trainer

What's a workout to make me look lean and tall?
—Stephen, Oak Park, IL

Posture is everything here. Strengthening your core will help you stand tall throughout the day. Do one or two sets of 10 to 15 repetitions of the front bridge, side bridge, and glute bridge every morning. Warm up first with forward and lateral lunges, hand walks, hip-flexor stretches, and chest stretches.

WEEK 34   WEEK OF / / TO / /   DAY:

STRENGTH TRAINING

EXERCISE	WEIGHT	WARMUP SETS			WORK SETS		
		SET 1 REPS	SET 2 REPS	SET 3 REPS	SET 1 REPS	SET 2 REPS	SET 3 REPS

NOTES: _____

CARDIO

TYPE	INTENSITY	DURATION

NOTES: _____

TRAINING TIP
STAY STRONG LONGER

Scientists have uncovered a new supplement that may help pack on muscle. In a recent report in *Strength and Conditioning Journal*, three recent studies show that the amino acid beta-alanine improves exercise performance. The mechanism? It helps ward off fatigue by improving a process known as carnosine synthesis. "Beta-alanine is where creatine was in 1992," says Jeffrey Stout, CSCS, PhD, author of the report. "A couple of studies showed potential, but not enough to make solid recommendations." In the next couple of years, more research will be published on beta-alanine to help determine whether the amino acid deserves its early praise, says Dr. Stout. Until then, he suggests sticking with proven muscle-building supplements, such as creatine and whey protein.

WEEK 34 | WEEK OF / / TO / / | DAY:

STRENGTH TRAINING

EXERCISE	WEIGHT	WARMUP SETS			WORK SETS		
		SET 1 REPS	SET 2 REPS	SET 3 REPS	SET 1 REPS	SET 2 REPS	SET 3 REPS

NOTES: _____

CARDIO

TYPE	INTENSITY	DURATION

NOTES: _____

163

SPOTLIGHT EXERCISE

BARBELL UPRIGHT ROW

The barbell upright row works all three portions of your deltoids (front, middle, and rear). It also involves the trapezius, biceps, lower back, and abdominal muscles. Perform two or three sets of 8 to 12 repetitions of the upright row near the end of your upper-body or shoulder routine.

Try to avoid common mistakes, which include leaning back as you pull the bar up, using a grip that's too wide or too narrow, and rushing the movement.

1. Stand with a barbell on the floor in front of you, your feet slightly less than shoulder-width apart. Grab the bar overhanded, your hands at shoulder width or slightly wider, and rest the bar on your thighs.

2. Draw the bar up toward your chin, keeping it close to your body. Go slowly and under control—take 3 seconds to lift the bar from your thighs to above your nipples.

3. Your elbows should remain flared outward during the movement. When the bar is above your nipples, pause for 2 seconds and contract your shoulders and trapezius.

4. Slowly lower the bar until your arms are straight, elbows unlocked.

WEEK 34 | **WEEK OF** / / **TO** / / | **DAY:**

STRENGTH TRAINING

EXERCISE	WEIGHT	WARM-UP SETS			WORK SETS		
		SET 1 REPS	SET 2 REPS	SET 3 REPS	SET 1 REPS	SET 2 REPS	SET 3 REPS

NOTES: _____

CARDIO

TYPE	INTENSITY	DURATION

NOTES: _____

TRAINING TIP

GET A GRIP ON A BETTER BENCH PRESS

The grip: Wide, overhand: Hands twice shoulder-width apart, palms facing forward

The benefit: Stresses the lower portion of the chest more than the other grips

The grip: Medium, overhand: Hands just beyond shoulder width, palms facing forward

The benefit: Places more emphasis on the triceps than a wide grip does

The grip: Narrow, overhand: Hands shoulder-width apart, palms facing forward

The benefit: Recruits the triceps more than the other grips do

The grip: Medium, underhand: Hands just beyond shoulder width, palms toward you

The benefit: Involves the biceps the most

The grip: Wide, underhand: Hands twice shoulder-width apart, palms toward you

The benefit: Works the upper portion of the chest best

WEEK 35 | WEEK OF / / TO / / | DAY:

STRENGTH TRAINING

EXERCISE	WEIGHT	WARMUP SETS			WORK SETS		
		SET 1 REPS	SET 2 REPS	SET 3 REPS	SET 1 REPS	SET 2 REPS	SET 3 REPS

NOTES: _____

CARDIO

TYPE	INTENSITY	DURATION

NOTES: _____

SCULPT AND STRENGTHEN

BOOST YOUR ENDURANCE

Adding the following plyometric exercises to your workout will help you run faster. Try the exercise below to improve your 5- or 10-K.

SIDE-TO-SIDE ANKLE HOP

With feet together, hop side to side (about 2 to 3 feet each way). Use only your ankles and calves. Do two sets of 15 explosive hops.

STANDING LONG JUMP

Dip into a quarter squat position. Push your arms back, then extend your lower body as you jump out and up. Do five sets of six jumps.

WEEK 35 WEEK OF / / TO / / DAY:

STRENGTH TRAINING

EXERCISE	WEIGHT	WARM-UP SETS						WORK SETS					
		SET 1		SET 2		SET 3		SET 1		SET 2		SET 3	
		REPS		REPS		REPS		REPS		REPS		REPS	

NOTES: _____

CARDIO

TYPE	INTENSITY	DURATION

NOTES: _____

Ask the Trainer

I'm training for a marathon and don't want to lose muscle. How can I preserve it?
—*Adam, Athens, GA*

Don't sweat it. You could do a couple of total-body workouts a week on off days, but lean mass means more work for your body when you run. That's why great marathoners have slight frames. Focus on nutrition, and warm up with exercises for hip and trunk stability, like lunges and crunches. When you've completed your marathon, hit the weights hard and your mass will jump right back.

WEEK 35 | WEEK OF / / TO / / | DAY:

STRENGTH TRAINING

EXERCISE	WEIGHT	WARMUP SETS			WORK SETS		
		SET 1 REPS	SET 2 REPS	SET 3 REPS	SET 1 REPS	SET 2 REPS	SET 3 REPS

NOTES:

CARDIO

TYPE	INTENSITY	DURATION

NOTES:

CORE POWER

TWISTING MEDICINE-BALL TOSS

Start this partner-assisted exercise lying flat on your back, knees bent. Your partner should stand a few feet in front of you and to your right. Curl up to catch a medicine ball he or she throws toward the left side of your body and slowly twist your body to your left, lowering your torso as you go. Touch the ball to the floor as your partner moves to your left. Curl yourself up and toss the ball back. Alternate sides and repeat 12 to 16 times in each direction. Perform three sets altogether.

WEEK 35 | WEEK OF / / TO / / | DAY:

STRENGTH TRAINING

EXERCISE	WEIGHT	WARMUP SETS			WORK SETS		
		SET 1 REPS	SET 2 REPS	SET 3 REPS	SET 1 REPS	SET 2 REPS	SET 3 REPS

NOTES:

CARDIO

TYPE	INTENSITY	DURATION

NOTES:

| WEEK 36 | WEEK OF / / TO / / | DAY: |

STRENGTH TRAINING

		WARMUP SETS			WORK SETS		
EXERCISE	WEIGHT	SET 1 REPS	SET 2 REPS	SET 3 REPS	SET 1 REPS	SET 2 REPS	SET 3 REPS

NOTES: _____

CARDIO

TYPE	INTENSITY	DURATION

NOTES: _____

FUELING UP

WAKE UP RIGHT

This healthy take on French toast is a great breakfast. The protein powder in the batter is exactly what your muscles crave after a night's fast, and the fruit topping won't spike your blood sugar the way most syrups will.

Muscle Toast

2 scoops vanilla whey-protein powder

½ teaspoon cinnamon

4 eggs (2 whole eggs and 2 egg whites)

⅓ cup fat-free milk

4 slices 100% whole-wheat bread

Fruit Topping

1 ripe banana, mashed

1 tablespoon whole-fruit strawberry preserves

1 tablespoon water

In a large bowl, mix the protein powder, cinnamon, eggs, and milk. Whisk until blended. Soak each slice of bread in the egg-and-protein mixture for 30 seconds. Spray a non-stick pan with cooking spray and cook each side on medium to medium-high heat until slightly firm. Mash the banana and mix it with the preserves and water. Top the toast with the fruit mixture.

BODY MOVING

BANISH LOWER-BACK PAIN

Pro cyclists make their living with their legs, but when the road turns rough, the lower back pays the bills. "As soon as your back starts fatiguing in a race, you lose efficiency, and you can't take advantage of the power in your legs," says George Hincapie, the reigning USPRO road-racing champ. Take a page from Hincapie's spine-fortification plan with a simple exercise called bird dogs. On all fours, with your knees directly below your hips and your hands directly below your shoulders, raise your right arm and your left leg and hold them parallel to the floor for 2 seconds. Lower them and alternate arms and legs. Start with three sets of 10 to 15 repetitions.

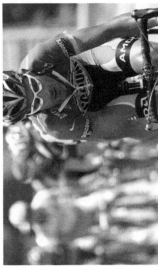

| WEEK 36 | WEEK OF / / TO / / | DAY: |

STRENGTH TRAINING

EXERCISE	WEIGHT	WARMUP SETS						WORK SETS					
		SET 1		SET 2		SET 3		SET 1		SET 2		SET 3	
		REPS		REPS		REPS		REPS		REPS		REPS	

NOTES:

CARDIO

TYPE	INTENSITY	DURATION

NOTES:

Ask the Trainer

Will running when my legs are still sore from a workout hurt my strength gains?
—*Theo, Jackson, TN*

If you're beginning a workout program, your legs may be sore from new stress. If running is part of your first week's plan, it's fine to work through the soreness; but if you're still hurting after a week, stop running. Instead, rest more between workouts. That said, long, slow distance runs hurt your strength gains, whether you're sore or not. Sprints and intervals complement strength training while improving your cardiovascular system.

| WEEK 36 | WEEK OF / / TO / / | DAY: |

STRENGTH TRAINING

EXERCISE	WEIGHT	WARMUP SETS			WORK SETS		
		SET 1 REPS	SET 2 REPS	SET 3 REPS	SET 1 REPS	SET 2 REPS	SET 3 REPS

NOTES:

CARDIO

TYPE	INTENSITY	DURATION

NOTES:

FUELING UP
QUICK FOOD FIXES

You don't have to braise, poach, or glaze food to make it tasty. But even simple meals can be screwed up. Four tips from Alton Brown, host, writer, and director of *Good Eats* and author of *Gear for Your Kitchen*.

Pasta. Use at least a gallon of water to let the noodles shake off starch. Salt the water—at least 1 tablespoon per gallon—for seasoning. Once it's boiling, add 1 teaspoon of oil to increase surface tension and keep the pot from boiling over.

Not-hard-boiled eggs. Put them in a steamer; it's gentle- and faster than boiling—12 minutes for as many as six eggs. When they're done, put them in ice-cold water and shell them right away. You'll get delicate whites and set yolks that aren't racquetball-hard.

Fish. Broiling minimizes fish funk, and some spices deodorize. Go with salmon, brush it with olive oil, and sprinkle on cumin, chili powder, and coriander—no pepper; pepper burns. Put it 4 inches under the broiler for 5 minutes. Forget flipping. Feel it to see if it's done—firm with a little bounce. Variation throughout the fish is fine, but if the grain separates, it's overdone.

WEEK 36 | WEEK OF / / TO / / | DAY:

STRENGTH TRAINING

EXERCISE	WEIGHT	WARMUP SETS			WORK SETS		
		SET 1 REPS	SET 2 REPS	SET 3 REPS	SET 1 REPS	SET 2 REPS	SET 3 REPS

NOTES:

CARDIO

TYPE	INTENSITY	DURATION

NOTES:

SPOTLIGHT EXERCISE

MEDICINE-BALL ARCHBISHOP

Place three to five medicine balls in a semicircle and assume the pushup position with both hands on the ball to the far left. Your chest should be over the ball and your feet should remain in place throughout the exercise.

Move your right hand to the ball at right and do a pushup. Bring your left hand to that ball.

Continue moving right and doing pushups until you reach the farthest ball. Then work your way back. That's one repetition.

| WEEK 37 | WEEK OF / / TO / / | DAY: |

STRENGTH TRAINING

EXERCISE	WEIGHT	WARMUP SETS			WORK SETS		
		SET 1 REPS	SET 2 REPS	SET 3 REPS	SET 1 REPS	SET 2 REPS	SET 3 REPS

NOTES:

CARDIO

TYPE	INTENSITY	DURATION

NOTES:

FUELING UP
CAN THE ENERGY DRINKS

Is your diet leaving you sluggish? Make sure you opt for a sugar-free pick-me-up. New Zealand scientists discovered that many popular energy drinks are worse for your gut than soda is, despite claiming to boost your metabolism. Why? They're often packed with sugar. The researchers observed that downing an energy drink containing 80 milligrams of caffeine and 24 grams of sugar—about the amount in an 8.3-ounce can of Red Bull—completely inhibited people's ability to burn fat. While caffeine does help speed metabolism, combining it with sugar negates its short-term fat-burning benefits, says lead author Elaine Rush, PhD.

WEEK 37 | **WEEK OF / / TO / /** | **DAY:**

STRENGTH TRAINING

EXERCISE	WEIGHT	WARMUP SETS			WORK SETS		
		SET 1 REPS	SET 2 REPS	SET 3 REPS	SET 1 REPS	SET 2 REPS	SET 3 REPS

NOTES: _____

CARDIO

TYPE	INTENSITY	DURATION

NOTES: _____

SCULPT AND STRENGTHEN

EASY SET, HARD BODY

Add a light set to the end of your strength workout. In a study in the *Journal of Strength and Conditioning Research*, Japanese researchers found that your body will pump out more growth hormone if you finish your heavy-weight-lifting session with a single, high-repetition set of an exercise using light weight. "This could be partially responsible for greater strength gains," says Kazushige Goto, PhD, the study's lead author. A typical strength workout might be five sets at 90 percent of your one-rep max, followed by 20 reps at 50 percent of your one-rep max.

| WEEK 37 | WEEK OF / / TO / / | DAY: |

STRENGTH TRAINING

EXERCISE	WEIGHT	WARMUP SETS			WORK SETS		
		SET 1	SET 2	SET 3	SET 1	SET 2	SET 3
		REPS	REPS	REPS	REPS	REPS	REPS

NOTES: _____

CARDIO

TYPE	INTENSITY	DURATION

NOTES: _____

ZINC IS FOR ZOOM

In the alphabet soup of vitamins and minerals, don't forget zinc. Zinc helps you maintain your energy level, according to research in the *American Journal of Clinical Nutrition*. In a 2-year study, 14 men either consumed 3.5 milligrams of zinc through their daily diets or took a 15-milligram zinc supplement. When tested on a stationary bike, those with the extra zinc could go hard longer and had lower heart rates and greater VO_2 max. The study's author, Henry Lukaski, PhD, of the U.S. Department of Agriculture's Human Nutrition Research Center, says zinc fuels enzymes in your red blood cells that clear out excess carbon dioxide during exercise. Nearly 20 percent of men don't take in the recommended 11 milligrams per day, so look to fortified cereals, beans, and lean red meat. Or take a multivitamin, which will give you an easy 15 milligrams.

WEEK 37 | **WEEK OF** / / **TO** / / | **DAY:**

STRENGTH TRAINING

EXERCISE	WEIGHT	WARMUP SETS			WORK SETS		
		SET 1 REPS	SET 2 REPS	SET 3 REPS	SET 1 REPS	SET 2 REPS	SET 3 REPS

NOTES: _____

CARDIO

TYPE	INTENSITY	DURATION

NOTES: _____

Ask the Trainer

My knees take a pounding when I play sports. Any strategies to keep them healthy?

—P.P., Flint, MI

Work on your landings. Whether you're jumping on a basketball court or bounding across a tennis court, your knees are at risk if you don't have the strength to decelerate the load—that load being you.

"I don't think there's enough emphasis placed on our ability to bring our bodies to a controlled stop," says Robert dos Remedios, CSCS, MA, director of speed, strength, and conditioning at the College of the Canyons, in Santa Clarita, California. If you plan on doing any type of explosive training—the kind needed for most sports—make landings part of your workouts for at least a month, says dos Remedios.

Between sets of squats or other leg exercises, do five jumps on a semisoft surface, like a rubber-matted area in your gym. Stand with your feet shoulder-width apart. Jump straight up. Then focus on landing with your knees bent, your shoulders slightly forward, and your butt and hips back. Try to land on the front two-thirds of your feet.

WEEK 38   WEEK OF / / TO / /   DAY:

STRENGTH TRAINING

EXERCISE	WEIGHT	WARMUP SETS			WORK SETS		
		SET 1 REPS	SET 2 REPS	SET 3 REPS	SET 1 REPS	SET 2 REPS	SET 3 REPS

NOTES: _____

CARDIO

TYPE	INTENSITY	DURATION

NOTES: _____

TRAINING TIP

Hit a plateau with the amount of weight you can squat? Once a week after your squat routine, perform three sets of 20 reps of the Hatfield back raise.

HATFIELD BACK RAISE

Kneel beside a weight bench. Bend forward at the waist so your stomach rests on the bench and hold a light weight plate behind your head. Contract your abs, relax your back, and lower your shoulders toward the floor. Without changing your hip angle, squeeze your lower-back muscles to lift your body back up. Do three or four sets of six to eight reps.

WEEK 38   WEEK OF / / TO / /   DAY:

STRENGTH TRAINING

EXERCISE	WEIGHT	WARMUP SETS						WORK SETS					
		SET 1		SET 2		SET 3		SET 1		SET 2		SET 3	
		REPS		REPS		REPS		REPS		REPS		REPS	

NOTES:

CARDIO

TYPE	INTENSITY	DURATION

NOTES:

Ask the Trainer

If I've had only a few hours of sleep, should I force myself to go to the gym, or skip it?
—*Jim, Temple, TX*

Take a pass. You don't need the added stress of a workout. Stress is cumulative—whether it's put on your body through training or by the demands of work and relationships. Remember, the goal of training should be to optimize health over a lifetime—elite bodies aren't built in a day. Manage your workouts based on long-term perspective, not short-term insecurity.

| WEEK 38 | WEEK OF / / TO / / | DAY: |

STRENGTH TRAINING

EXERCISE	WEIGHT	WARMUP SETS			WORK SETS		
		SET 1 REPS	SET 2 REPS	SET 3 REPS	SET 1 REPS	SET 2 REPS	SET 3 REPS

NOTES:

CARDIO

TYPE	INTENSITY	DURATION

NOTES:

TRAINING TIP
BE A SUPER DAD

Here's a great two-fer: Be a good dad and get a good workout. Playing with your kids can be as beneficial as certain workouts, according to a new study in the *Journal of Sports Medicine and Physical Fitness*. Just 20 minutes of playing soccer and dodgeball raised adults' heartbeats to 88 percent of their maximum and burned 160 calories, researchers found; half an hour burned 240 calories—about the same as a moderate bike ride. The games were more than enough "to produce training effects and benefits from physical activity," says study coauthor Phillip Watts, PhD, of Northern Michigan University in Marquette.

WEEK 38 | WEEK OF / / TO / / | DAY:

STRENGTH TRAINING

EXERCISE	WEIGHT	WARMUP SETS			WORK SETS		
		SET 1 REPS	SET 2 REPS	SET 3 REPS	SET 1 REPS	SET 2 REPS	SET 3 REPS

NOTES:

CARDIO

TYPE	INTENSITY	DURATION

NOTES:

FITNESS FACT

WARNING: LABELS

Eating low-fat foods may be making you fat. Cornell University researchers discovered that when overweight people thought they were eating low-fat M&Ms, they consumed 47 percent more calories than those who were given regular M&Ms. But the only difference between the candies was the label—there's no such thing as a low-fat version of the product. "People typically underestimate the calories that a low-fat snack contains, saying it has about 40 percent fewer calories than it actually does," says study author Brian Wansink, PhD. On average, however, low-fat foods contain just 15 percent fewer calories than full-fat products do. Since most people rate low-fat foods as less tasty and satisfying, Dr. Wansink has a simple suggestion: "Stick with the regular food you like, but eat a smaller amount."

WEEK 39	WEEK OF / / TO / /	DAY:

STRENGTH TRAINING

EXERCISE	WEIGHT	WARMUP SETS						WORK SETS					
		SET 1		SET 2		SET 3		SET 1		SET 2		SET 3	
		REPS		REPS		REPS		REPS		REPS		REPS	

NOTES:

CARDIO

TYPE	INTENSITY	DURATION

NOTES:

STRETCH IT OUT

BENT-OVER TWIST

This stretch does wonders for range of motion and flexibility in your trunk and hips.

Stand with your feet wider than shoulder-width apart. Place your left hand on your right ankle (or right knee if you can't reach that far). Raise your right arm straight up so your hand is pointing at the ceiling. Hold this position for 3 to 5 seconds, then rotate your trunk and place your right hand on your left ankle or knee, pointing your left arm straight up. Rotate back and forth five to 10 times.

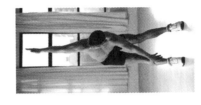

WEEK 39 | WEEK OF / / TO / / | DAY:

STRENGTH TRAINING

EXERCISE	WEIGHT	WARMUP SETS						WORK SETS					
		SET 1		SET 2		SET 3		SET 1		SET 2		SET 3	
		REPS		REPS		REPS		REPS		REPS		REPS	

NOTES:

CARDIO

TYPE	INTENSITY	DURATION

NOTES:

PET PROJECT

There's scientific proof that people look like their dogs: A recent study found that when both people and pets went on a diet and took walks together, both lost weight. Take General Patton on a stroll farther than the backyard to do his business. If you're canine deficient, adopt a best friend. Or offer to walk your cute neighbor's pooch. You dog, you.

WEEK 39   WEEK OF / / TO / /   DAY:

STRENGTH TRAINING

EXERCISE	WEIGHT	WARMUP SETS			WORK SETS		
		SET 1 REPS	SET 2 REPS	SET 3 REPS	SET 1 REPS	SET 2 REPS	SET 3 REPS

NOTES:

CARDIO

TYPE	INTENSITY	DURATION

NOTES:

TRAINING TIP
BREATHE LIKE A YOGI

Gumby limbs and inner peace are fine, but new research also shows that yoga training helps you breathe better by expanding lung capacity. Researchers at Thailand's Khon Kaen University had 29 volunteers participate in 20-minute yoga sessions three times a week for 6 weeks. Compared with a control group, the yoga crowd significantly increased total chest-wall expansion and exhalation volume, "allowing individuals to get more air to the base of the lung," the researchers report. The result is more oxygen with each breath and less effort to breathe.

| WEEK 39 | WEEK OF / / TO / / | DAY: |

STRENGTH TRAINING

EXERCISE	WEIGHT	WARM-UP SETS						WORK SETS					
		SET 1		SET 2		SET 3		SET 1		SET 2		SET 3	
		REPS		REPS		REPS		REPS		REPS		REPS	

NOTES: _____

CARDIO

TYPE	INTENSITY	DURATION

NOTES: _____

| WEEK 40 | WEEK OF / / TO / / | DAY: |

STRENGTH TRAINING

		WARMUP SETS			WORK SETS		
		SET 1	SET 2	SET 3	SET 1	SET 2	SET 3
EXERCISE	WEIGHT	REPS	REPS	REPS	REPS	REPS	REPS

NOTES: _____

CARDIO

TYPE	INTENSITY	DURATION

NOTES: _____

FUELING UP

THE CARB CUTOFF

Are you in the fat-burning zone? University of Florida scientists recently determined that dieters who eat less than 100 grams of carbohydrates daily lose an average of 4 pounds more fat a month than those whose carb intake is higher. The discovery was made when researchers analyzed 87 weight-loss studies comparing a variety of carbohydrate intakes, varying from 1 percent to 75 percent of the total calories consumed. One likely mechanism for the benefit: "As carbohydrate intake goes down, so do levels of insulin—a hormone that signals your body to store fat," says lead investigator James Krieger, MS. For reference, one slice of whole-grain bread, or ½ cup of cooked pasta or rice, packs 15 to 20 grams of carbohydrates; 1 cup of high-fiber vegetables—such as broccoli, cauliflower, or green beans—has about 6 grams; an 8-ounce glass of milk contains 12 grams; and a regular 12-ounce beer contains 13 grams.

Ask the Trainer

My shoulders pop when I lift weights—no matter how much weight I use. Should I be worried?
—Jason, Miami, FL

It's like clicking in the knee or elbow—in most cases, nothing's wrong. The sound is likely caused by soft-tissue movement or improper displacement of the limbs at the elbow joint. You should have a trainer check your form, and if you feel pain or find that your range of motion is limited, stop and check with a physician

WEEK 40	WEEK OF / / TO / /	DAY:

STRENGTH TRAINING

EXERCISE	WEIGHT	WARMUP SETS						WORK SETS					
		SET 1		SET 2		SET 3		SET 1		SET 2		SET 3	
		REPS		REPS		REPS		REPS		REPS		REPS	

NOTES: _____

CARDIO

TYPE	INTENSITY	DURATION

NOTES: _____

| WEEK 40 | WEEK OF / / TO / / | DAY: |

TRAINING TIP

To get more defined pecs and that full-chest look, try the reverse pushup:

REVERSE PUSHUP

Lie under a barbell set in the supports of a squat rack. Grab the bar with your thumbs on the same side of the bar as your fingers and support your weight on the backs of your heels. Pull yourself up until your chest almost touches the bar. Hold this position for 3 seconds, then slowly lower yourself until your arms are straight. Do two or three sets of 6 to 10 reps.

STRENGTH TRAINING

| | | WARMUP SETS | | | WORK SETS | | |
EXERCISE	WEIGHT	SET 1 REPS	SET 2 REPS	SET 3 REPS	SET 1 REPS	SET 2 REPS	SET 3 REPS

NOTES:

CARDIO

TYPE	INTENSITY	DURATION

NOTES:

FUELING UP

CHAIN REACTION

Build muscle without breaking a sweat. University of West Florida scientists recently discovered that downing a sports drink with amino acids before you lift may make your workout easier. The researchers compared two sports drinks: one containing branched-chain amino acids (BCAA)—the proteins that are a major part of muscle tissue—and one without the added nutrients. The result: When the study subjects drank 16 ounces of the BCAA-infused drink before doing a set of bench presses, their perceived exertion declined by 16 percent, compared with that of men who consumed a regular sports drink. In the study, the scientists were testing a product called Amino Vital; you can find it at www.amino-vital.com or your local health food store.

| WEEK 40 | WEEK OF / / TO / / | DAY: |

STRENGTH TRAINING

EXERCISE	WEIGHT	WARMUP SETS						WORK SETS					
		SET 1		SET 2		SET 3		SET 1		SET 2		SET 3	
		REPS		REPS		REPS		REPS		REPS		REPS	

NOTES: _____

CARDIO

TYPE	INTENSITY	DURATION

NOTES: _____

WEEK OF   / /   TO   / /   DAY:

TRAINING TIP

POWER UP YOUR SWING

Working your back can build your chest. According to a new study by Australian researchers, performing a power exercise for one muscle group can increase power in the antagonistic—or opposite—muscle group. This principle can give you a pregame power boost, says study author Daniel Baker, CSCS. "For instance, baseball hitters and golfers can take practice swings as if they are lefties (if they're right-handed), and vice versa. Tennis players should warm up by swinging in each direction."

STRENGTH TRAINING

		WARMUP SETS			WORK SETS		
EXERCISE	WEIGHT	SET 1 REPS	SET 2 REPS	SET 3 REPS	SET 1 REPS	SET 2 REPS	SET 3 REPS

NOTES:

CARDIO

TYPE	INTENSITY	DURATION

NOTES:

FITNESS FACT

MORE MUSCLE, LESS TIME

The key to faster gains? Shorter workouts. Japanese researchers found that reducing your rest time between sets can cause your body to secrete more physique-enhancing hormones. In the study, men who rested 1 minute between sets of 10 repetitions exhibited higher blood levels of growth hormone—which signals your body to build muscle and burn fat—than those who completed the same amount of work in a longer period of time. This seemed to translate to better results: The men who kept their workouts moving gained more muscle and strength, and burned more fat, than the men whose lifting sessions lasted longer.

WEEK 41	WEEK OF / / TO / /	DAY:

STRENGTH TRAINING

EXERCISE	WEIGHT	WARM-UP SETS			WORK SETS		
		SET 1 REPS	SET 2 REPS	SET 3 REPS	SET 1 REPS	SET 2 REPS	SET 3 REPS

NOTES: _____

CARDIO

TYPE	INTENSITY	DURATION

NOTES: _____

FUELING UP

STEALTH HEALTH FOOD: KEFIR

Similar to yogurt, this fermented dairy beverage is made by culturing fresh milk with kefir grains. Because kefir contains gut-friendly bacteria, it's been shown to lower cholesterol, improve lactose digestion, and enhance the immune system. In addition, University of Washington scientists recently demonstrated that kefir was more effective than fruit juice or other dairy beverages at helping people control hunger. Look for kefir in the health food section of your local supermarket, or in the dairy isle of health food stores, such as Whole Foods.

WEEK 41	WEEK OF / / TO / /	DAY:

STRENGTH TRAINING

EXERCISE	WEIGHT	WARMUP SETS						WORK SETS					
		SET 1		SET 2		SET 3		SET 1		SET 2		SET 3	
		REPS		REPS		REPS		REPS		REPS		REPS	

NOTES:

CARDIO

TYPE	INTENSITY	DURATION

NOTES:

BODY MOVING

BREATHING LESSONS

Swim faster by breathing less? It's possible. A study found that swimmers who reduce the frequency of their breaths improve the delivery of oxygen to their muscles. Researchers at the University of the Pacific found that controlled-frequency breathing (CFB) provides the benefits of high-intensity training while the athlete swims at a moderate intensity. In the study, swimmers breathed after every eighth stroke rather than after the usual second or third stroke. "CFB improves oxygen extraction from the lungs," says study author Sharon West, PhD. Try it in your warmup or during long-distance swims.

WEEK 41 WEEK OF / / TO / / DAY:

STRENGTH TRAINING

EXERCISE	WEIGHT	WARMUP SETS			WORK SETS		
		SET 1 REPS	SET 2 REPS	SET 3 REPS	SET 1 REPS	SET 2 REPS	SET 3 REPS

NOTES:

CARDIO

TYPE	INTENSITY	DURATION

NOTES:

WEEK 42	WEEK OF / / TO / /	DAY:

STRENGTH TRAINING

EXERCISE	WEIGHT	WARMUP SETS						WORK SETS					
		SET 1		SET 2		SET 3		SET 1		SET 2		SET 3	
		REPS		REPS		REPS		REPS		REPS		REPS	

NOTES:

CARDIO

TYPE	INTENSITY	DURATION

NOTES:

BODY MOVING

LIFT YOUR HEART RATE

Get in your cardio while you lift. A study at the University of Hawaii found that circuit training with weights—performing one exercise after another without rest—raises your heart rate 15 beats per minute higher than running at about 60 to 70 percent of your maximum heart rate. According to the study, circuit training strengthens your muscles and provides cardiovascular benefits similar to those of aerobic exercise. The men in the study repeated circuits of 10 exercises for just less than 20 minutes, performing moves like bench presses, rows, and lat pulldowns with light resistance.

Ask the Trainer

What if I'm not hungry enough to eat several small meals a day to keep my metabolism up?
—Kevin, Nashville, TN

Don't skip meals. Rely on healthy snacks to bridge the gaps between meals (which may mean eating five or six times a day). And—this is crucial—obey your body's signals of hunger and fullness. The key is to avoid overeating, not to log a certain number of meals.

WEEK 42	WEEK OF / / TO / /	DAY:

STRENGTH TRAINING

EXERCISE	WEIGHT	WARM-UP SETS			WORK SETS		
		SET 1 REPS	SET 2 REPS	SET 3 REPS	SET 1 REPS	SET 2 REPS	SET 3 REPS

NOTES:

CARDIO

TYPE	INTENSITY	DURATION

NOTES:

FITNESS FACT
MEGADOSE DANGER

Here's proof that you can get too much of a good thing: British researchers discovered that high doses of vitamin C can slow muscle recovery. When healthy men took 1,000 milligrams (mg) of the vitamin daily, they experienced decreased muscle strength for a full week after intense running, compared with those who skipped the supplement. However, previous studies report that moderate intake of vitamin C—100 to 500 mg a day—speeds recovery. So why isn't more C better? The scientists suspect that the higher dose reduces the number of scavenger cells, which clean up debris from muscle damage and signal your body that your muscles need repair. Cap your supplementation at 500 mg a day, an amount a Japanese study found also reduces the frequency of colds.

WEEK 42 | WEEK OF / / TO / / | DAY:

EXERCISE	WEIGHT	WARMUP SETS						WORK SETS					
		SET 1 REPS	SET 2 REPS	SET 3 REPS	SET 1 REPS	SET 2 REPS	SET 3 REPS

NOTES: _____

CARDIO

TYPE	INTENSITY	DURATION

NOTES: _____

STRETCH IT OUT

INJURY-PROOF YOUR ABS

This exercise improves your ability to rotate your torso and extend your hips, while strengthening your abs and legs, which may help prevent a sports hernia.

REAR LUNGE WITH POSTERIOR LATERAL REACH

1. Stand holding a light dumbbell in front of your chest.

2. Step back with your left leg while raising the weight up and back over your right shoulder. Look at the weight as you move it up. Push yourself back up to the starting position. Do 10 to 12 repetitions, then repeat, this time lunging back with your right leg and bringing the weight over your left shoulder.

WEEK 42 WEEK OF / / TO / / DAY:

STRENGTH TRAINING

EXERCISE	WEIGHT	WARMUP SETS			WORK SETS		
		SET 1 REPS	SET 2 REPS	SET 3 REPS	SET 1 REPS	SET 2 REPS	SET 3 REPS

NOTES:

CARDIO

TYPE	INTENSITY	DURATION

NOTES:

FUELING UP

TEST YOUR CALORIE IQ

University of Arkansas researchers discovered that people underestimated the number of calories in restaurant meals by as much as 93 percent. Could you have done better? Check out the average guess—along with the actual calorie count—for three popular dishes.

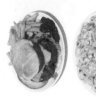
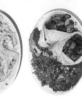

HAMBURGER AND FRIES

Average guess: 777
Actual number: 1,240

FETTUCCINE ALFREDO

Average guess: 704
Actual number: 1,500

CHICKEN FAJITAS

Average guess: 704
Actual number: 1,660

WEEK 43   WEEK OF / / TO / /   DAY:

STRENGTH TRAINING

EXERCISE	WEIGHT	WARMUP SETS			WORK SETS		
		SET 1 REPS	SET 2 REPS	SET 3 REPS	SET 1 REPS	SET 2 REPS	SET 3 REPS

NOTES: _____

CARDIO

TYPE	INTENSITY	DURATION

NOTES: _____

SCULPT AND STRENGTHEN

GAIN WITHOUT PAIN

To prevent shoulder pain, try these tweaks from the *Strength and Conditioning Journal.*

BENCH PRESS

To prevent your arms from going below shoulder height (which can strain your shoulders) place a rolled-up towel or your sternum to limit the bar's descent.

LAT PULLDOWN

Use an underhand grip, hands less than shoulder-width apart. Lean back slightly and, keeping your back straight, pull the bar toward your chest. Allow your arms to straighten to the starting position.

SQUAT

Hold the bar in the crooks of your fingers so it rests on the front of your shoulders, and keep your elbows high.

LATERAL RAISE

Hold dumbbells with thumbs up and your arms slightly in front of you to reduce rotator cuff stress.

WEEK 43		WEEK OF / / TO / /		DAY:

STRENGTH TRAINING

EXERCISE	WEIGHT	WARMUP SETS						WORK SETS					
		SET 1		SET 2		SET 3		SET 1		SET 2		SET 3	
		REPS		REPS		REPS		REPS		REPS		REPS	

NOTES:

CARDIO

TYPE	INTENSITY	DURATION

NOTES:

Ask the Trainer

Are situps bad for my back?
—Lance, Lansing, MI

Depends on what other exercises you do. If situps are a huge part of your workout, you'll find that your hip flexors—which go from the front of each thighbone through your abdominal cavity and attach to your spine—become increasingly tight. And tight hip flexors will pull on your lower back, causing pain. Stretching your hip flexors between sets and on the following day can help. But I strongly encourage you to focus on moves like Swiss-ball crunches, Russian twists, and front bridges, which strengthen your abs better than traditional situps without placing as much stress on your hip flexors.

WEEK 43 | **WEEK OF / / TO / /** | **DAY:**

STRENGTH TRAINING

EXERCISE	WEIGHT	WARMUP SETS			WORK SETS		
		SET 1 REPS	SET 2 REPS	SET 3 REPS	SET 1 REPS	SET 2 REPS	SET 3 REPS

NOTES:

CARDIO

TYPE	INTENSITY	DURATION

NOTES:

| WEEK 43 | WEEK OF / / TO / / | DAY: |

STRENGTH TRAINING

EXERCISE	WEIGHT	WARMUP SETS			WORK SETS		
		SET 1 REPS	SET 2 REPS	SET 3 REPS	SET 1 REPS	SET 2 REPS	SET 3 REPS

NOTES: _____

CARDIO

TYPE	INTENSITY	DURATION

NOTES: _____

FUELING UP
BE A BIG SUCK-UP

Catching your breath after a hard run just got a little easier. New Zealand scientists recently discovered that the more vitamin D in your system, the better your lungs function. "The difference in respiration between having high and low blood levels of vitamin D is more pronounced than that between former smokers and nonsmokers," says study author Peter Black, MD. The scientists believe that vitamin D may enhance tissue remodeling in the lungs, a biological process that occurs throughout life but declines with age. You need at least 20 micrograms of vitamin D per day, and if you're over 50, the amount doubles. Since fortified milk and seafood are the only viable food sources—each provides about half of your daily requirement per serving—you may want to consider a supplement. Look for one that contains D3 (cholecalciferol)—such as Carlson Laboratories' vitamin D gelcaps (www.carlsonlabs.com)—the most active form of the vitamin.

STRETCH IT OUT

DYNAMIC STRETCHING PREPS YOUR BODY AND BRAIN FOR ACTION

Try this stretch, called the pogo squat, from Blair O'Donovan, CSCS, sports-conditioning director at Elite Athlete Training Systems in Maryland, before any lower-body workout. It'll loosen your quads, hamstrings, and glutes, and increase bloodflow to your entire lower body.

POGO SQUAT

Stand with your feet about shoulder-width apart, arms hanging at your sides. Squat quickly until your thighs are almost parallel to the floor. Without pausing, jump as high as you can. Land softly, and immediately squat into the next repetition. Do 15 to 20 repetitions.

WEEK 44 | WEEK OF / / TO / / | DAY:

STRENGTH TRAINING

EXERCISE	WEIGHT	WARMUP SETS			WORK SETS		
		SET 1 REPS	SET 2 REPS	SET 3 REPS	SET 1 REPS	SET 2 REPS	SET 3 REPS

NOTES:

CARDIO

TYPE	INTENSITY	DURATION

NOTES:

Ask the Trainer

I'm bored with my abs routine. How can I shake it up?
—*Cliff, Atlanta, GA*

Use your Spidey sense. "The spider lift works on several planes of motion, especially the transverse, or diagonal, plane," says C. J. Murphy, MFS, owner of Total Performance Sports in Everett, Massachusetts. Most abdominal exercises crunch your torso forward or bring your legs up toward your chest, ignoring rotation and stabilization. This lift builds torso strength and stability and develops the quadratus lumborum, a muscle—close to the spine—that helps guard against back pain.

1. Grab a pair of dumbbells with palms toward your thighs and stand with your knees soft and your feet more than shoulder-width apart. Extend your left arm overhead, keeping your right arm at your side. Rotate your right hip back and your left hip forward, and look up at the dumbbell overhead.

2. Lower the weight in your right hand straight down as far as you can. As you go, push your hips back and allow your knees to bend slightly. Perform 8 to 10 reps, then reverse the movement so your right hand is overhead and your right hip is forward. Do another 8 to 10 reps in this position.

WEEK 44   WEEK OF / / TO / /   DAY:

STRENGTH TRAINING

EXERCISE	WEIGHT	WARMUP SETS			WORK SETS		
		SET 1 REPS	SET 2 REPS	SET 3 REPS	SET 1 REPS	SET 2 REPS	SET 3 REPS

NOTES:

CARDIO

TYPE	INTENSITY	DURATION

NOTES:

| WEEK 44 | WEEK OF / / TO / / | DAY: |

STRENGTH TRAINING

EXERCISE	WEIGHT	WARMUP SETS						WORK SETS					
		SET 1		SET 2		SET 3		SET 1		SET 2		SET 3	
		REPS		REPS		REPS		REPS		REPS		REPS	

NOTES: _____

CARDIO

TYPE	INTENSITY	DURATION

NOTES: _____

FUELING UP

THE THERMOGENIC DIET

Despite what many nutritionists say, all calories are not created equal. "The calorie-is-a-calorie theory takes into account the total energy in a food but ignores the energy that's required to process it," says Cassandra Forsythe, MS, a nutrition researcher at the University of Connecticut in Storrs. Case in point: Up to 30 percent of the calories in protein are burned through the digestive process, compared with just 8 percent of those in carbohydrates, and 2 percent of those in fat. Interestingly, alcohol tops the list, at 35 percent. This is known as the thermic effect of food; check out the examples below to see how it can dramatically impact your "actual" calorie intake.

CHICKEN MARSALA, COOKED SPINACH, AND GLASS OF WINE: 76 g protein, 12 g carbs, 9 g fat, 15 g alcohol

TOTAL CALORIES: 590; THERMIC EFFECT: 30%;
ACTUAL CALORIES: 413

PENNE ALFREDO, STEAMED BROCCOLI, AND GLASS OF BEER: 15 g protein, 61 g carbs, 20 g fat, 15 g alcohol

TOTAL CALORIES: 588; THERMIC EFFECT: 13%;
ACTUAL CALORIES: 511

HAMSTRING HELPER

You may think of hamstrings as the keys to speed. But it's important to train your hamstrings for deceleration to prevent injury. According to a recent essay in the *Strength and Conditioning Journal*, deceleration exercises strengthen the hamstrings and prepare them for the moment when the heel strikes the ground—the point at which most hamstring tears occur. Use this deceleration exercise from author Rob Vorhees, CSCS: On a seated-leg-curl machine, adjust the starting position so your knees are unable to hyperextend at the top of the movement. Set the resistance at 50 percent of your body weight. Keeping your spine in a neutral position, let your legs straighten as fast as possible and suddenly stop them just before the weight stack would hit bottom. Do three sets of 8 to 12 repetitions.

WEEK 44 WEEK OF / / TO / /   DAY:

STRENGTH TRAINING

EXERCISE	WEIGHT	WARMUP SETS						WORK SETS					
		SET 1		SET 2		SET 3		SET 1		SET 2		SET 3	
		REPS		REPS		REPS		REPS		REPS		REPS	

NOTES:

CARDIO

TYPE	INTENSITY	DURATION

NOTES:

| WEEK 45 | WEEK OF / / TO / / | DAY: |

FUELING UP

A GROWING PROBLEM

Want more proof that eating too many carbohydrates leads directly to weight gain? Check out the graph below:

Over the last 40 years, carb intake has risen by 33 percent; obesity has doubled.

Using data from the Centers for Disease Control and Prevention for the years 1960 through 1997, it shows how Americans' increasing intake of carbs coincides with a rise in obesity. Not shown: the incidence of diabetes also rising, by 47 percent.

STRENGTH TRAINING

EXERCISE	WEIGHT	WARMUP SETS						WORK SETS					
		SET 1		SET 2		SET 3		SET 1		SET 2		SET 3	
		REPS		REPS		REPS		REPS		REPS		REPS	

NOTES:

CARDIO

TYPE	INTENSITY	DURATION

NOTES:

Ask the Trainer

The harder my workout, the larger my appetite. Is it okay to pig out, since my body's in fat-burning mode?
—*Bill, Durango, CO*

No. Your body does need carbs and protein within 15 minutes of your last rep—but spreading out your eating will make better use of your elevated metabolism. Overloading your fat-burning engine can shunt extra calories to fat reserves.

WEEK 45 | **WEEK OF / / TO / /** | **DAY:**

STRENGTH TRAINING

EXERCISE	WEIGHT	WARMUP SETS			WORK SETS		
		SET 1 REPS	SET 2 REPS	SET 3 REPS	SET 1 REPS	SET 2 REPS	SET 3 REPS

NOTES:

CARDIO

TYPE	INTENSITY	DURATION

NOTES:

TRAINING TIP

SAVE THE CHEST FOR LAST

Move the chest fly to the end of your workout. When Truman State University researchers measured how hard muscles work during a barbell bench press, dumbbell bench press, and chest fly, they found that the barbell bench press is best for developing a bigger, stronger chest. The pectorals of the men and women in the study were activated for 23 percent less time during the chest fly, compared with the barbell bench press—and researchers didn't even measure the lowering phase of the lifts. The researchers say that dumbbell and barbell presses can be used interchangeably, but the chest fly should not be one of your primary lifts.

WEEK 45 | WEEK OF / / TO / / | DAY:

STRENGTH TRAINING

EXERCISE	WEIGHT	WARMUP SETS			WORK SETS		
		SET 1 REPS	SET 2 REPS	SET 3 REPS	SET 1 REPS	SET 2 REPS	SET 3 REPS

NOTES:

CARDIO

TYPE	INTENSITY	DURATION

NOTES:

Ask the Trainer

I started lifting weights 4 months ago and gained 10 pounds in the first 3 months. Then, nothing. What happened?

—Jerry, San Antonio, TX

Your body wised up and adapted to the punishment. To keep growing, start building muscle outside the gym—with nutrition and lifestyle choices. Bolster your workout with small meals or snacks before and after, and continue to eat frequently throughout the day. In the weight room, for 3 weeks make your sets last longer than 40 seconds (to gain size), then keep them under 25 seconds for the next 3 weeks (to build strength). Continue to alternate between these approaches, and you'll soon break out of that holding pattern.

| WEEK 45 | WEEK OF / / TO / / | DAY: |

STRENGTH TRAINING

EXERCISE	WEIGHT	WARM-UP SETS			WORK SETS		
		SET 1 REPS	SET 2 REPS	SET 3 REPS	SET 1 REPS	SET 2 REPS	SET 3 REPS

NOTES:

CARDIO

TYPE	INTENSITY	DURATION

NOTES:

WEEK 46

WEEK OF / / TO / / DAY:

STRENGTH TRAINING

EXERCISE	WEIGHT	WARMUP SETS			WORK SETS		
		SET 1 REPS	SET 2 REPS	SET 3 REPS	SET 1 REPS	SET 2 REPS	SET 3 REPS

NOTES:

CARDIO

TYPE	INTENSITY	DURATION

NOTES:

FUELING UP
NUKE YOUR GUT

It could be the coolest diet ever. Researchers at the University of Illinois recently found that frozen dinners may help speed weight loss. When scientists placed two groups of men on a 1,700-calorie diet for 8 weeks, they found that those who ate one-serving packaged meals for lunch and dinner lost 45 percent more weight than men who made their own meals. "People tend to think a healthy portion is larger than it really is, which probably explains the difference between groups," says lead author Sandra Hannum, MS, RD. The biggest losers ate Uncle Ben's bowls, which typically contain 350 to 400 calories per package. Want more variety? Check product labels for frozen entrées that have a similar number of calories and at least 20 grams of protein.

Ask the Trainer

Why does a tough workout make me nauseated?
—Jared, Maple Grove, MN

Push your body too hard and it will conserve energy by slowing the digestive process. So anything you ate or drank in the few hours before your workout will slosh around in your abdomen and cause a wave of nausea. "Usually people who feel sick when they exercise aren't in good physical condition to start with," says Steven Devor, PhD, a professor of exercise science at Ohio State University. So if you feel like heaving, slow your pace or rest more between sets. Once your stomach settles, gradually amp up your efforts. And don't slug sports drinks: They take longer to digest than water does.

WEEK 46 | WEEK OF / / TO / / | DAY:

STRENGTH TRAINING

EXERCISE	WEIGHT	WARMUP SETS						WORK SETS					
		SET 1		SET 2		SET 3		SET 1		SET 2		SET 3	
		REPS	REPS	REPS	REPS	REPS	REPS	REPS	REPS	REPS	REPS	REPS	REPS

NOTES:

CARDIO

TYPE	INTENSITY	DURATION

NOTES:

TRAINING TIP
THE NEW WARMUP

THE PELICAN WALK

Dynamic stretches—those that involve movement—prep your body and brain, flooding your muscles with blood and engaging your nervous system's muscular-control mechanisms. This one will loosen your hamstrings. Start by balancing on your left leg. With both hands, slowly reach down toward your left foot while your right leg rises straight back. You'll feel a stretch in your left hamstring. Return to the starting position, then step back and balance on your right leg while lifting your left leg straight back. Perform 12 to 14 repetitions.

WEEK 46 | **WEEK OF** / / **TO** / / | **DAY:**

STRENGTH TRAINING

EXERCISE	WEIGHT	WARMUP SETS						WORK SETS					
		SET 1		SET 2		SET 3		SET 1		SET 2		SET 3	
		REPS	REPS	REPS	REPS	REPS	REPS	REPS	REPS	REPS	REPS	REPS	REPS

NOTES:

CARDIO

TYPE	INTENSITY	DURATION

NOTES:

Ask the Trainer

How can I stop my postwork food cravings?
—Kevin, Chicago, IL

Worker bees eat lunch around 12:00 or 1:00 p.m., but dinner might not come until 8:00 p.m. A snack will blunt the craving and allow for a sensible dinner without the junk-food binge. My advice is to eat better earlier in the day (but don't gorge) and take advantage of a mid-afternoon break to down a quick snack, such as yogurt, ar. apple with a thin layer of peanut butter, or some string cheese.

WEEK 46 WEEK OF / / TO / / DAY:

STRENGTH TRAINING

EXERCISE	WEIGHT	WARMUP SETS			WORK SETS		
		SET 1	SET 2	SET 3	SET 1	SET 2	SET 3
		REPS	REPS	REPS	REPS	REPS	REPS

NOTES:

CARDIO

TYPE	INTENSITY	DURATION

NOTES:

SCULPT AND STRENGTHEN

TRICK OUT YOUR TRICEPS

For strength, power, endurance, and balance, try the triceps power pushup. Place a large medicine ball under your chest. Bend your arms to lower your chest to the ball. Push up forcefully so that your hands leave the floor, then land with your hands on the ball. Straighten your arms. Do a pushup with your hands on the ball, then drop your hands to the floor and repeat. Aim for three sets of 8 to 12 reps.

WEEK 47 WEEK OF / / TO / / DAY:

STRENGTH TRAINING

EXERCISE	WEIGHT	WARMUP SETS			WORK SETS		
		SET 1 REPS	SET 2 REPS	SET 3 REPS	SET 1 REPS	SET 2 REPS	SET 3 REPS

NOTES:

CARDIO

TYPE	INTENSITY	DURATION

NOTES:

FUELING UP

FRUIT FIGHTS FLAB

Here's scientific evidence that one weird diet might actually work. Louisiana State University researchers recently discovered that people who ate half a grapefruit three times a day lost 4 pounds in 12 weeks, even though they hadn't deliberately altered any other part of their diets. They also lowered their blood pressure by 6 points, enough to reduce their risk of stroke by 40 percent. Although the mechanism isn't clear, researchers speculate that grapefruit's acidity may slow your rate of digestion, helping keep you full longer. The scientists note that for weight loss, substituting 8 ounces of juice for each serving of the fruit is just as effective. Try Tropicana Pure Premium Ruby Red Grapefruit Juice: A new study determined that it contains more heart-healthy antioxidants than any other brand tested.

| WEEK 47 | WEEK OF / / TO / / | DAY: |

STRENGTH TRAINING

EXERCISE	WEIGHT	WARM-UP SETS			WORK SETS		
		SET 1 REPS	SET 2 REPS	SET 3 REPS	SET 1 REPS	SET 2 REPS	SET 3 REPS

NOTES: _____

CARDIO

TYPE	INTENSITY	DURATION

NOTES: _____

CORE POWER

WALK THIS WAY

Add some weight to your treadmill workout for a stronger core. According to a report published in the *Strength and Conditioning Journal*, building a muscle group called the gluteus medius/minimus (GMM) can improve your balance and core stability. The GMM is the muscle at the top of your butt, at your hip. A weak GMM "can predispose a person to lower-back pain," says Eric Wilson, CSCS, PT, author of the report. To strengthen your GMM, walk on a treadmill while holding a light dumbbell in one hand. Use a weight that's 5 to 15 percent of your body weight (e.g., a 180-pound man could use a 10-pound dumbbell), and switch the weight to your other hand halfway through your session.

| WEEK 47 | WEEK OF / / TO / / | DAY: |

STRENGTH TRAINING

EXERCISE	WEIGHT	WARMUP SETS			WORK SETS		
		SET 1 REPS	SET 2 REPS	SET 3 REPS	SET 1 REPS	SET 2 REPS	SET 3 REPS

NOTES: _____

CARDIO

TYPE	INTENSITY	DURATION

NOTES: _____

FITNESS FACT
REACH THE RIM

Improve your sports performance. In a study published in the *Journal of Strength and Conditioning Research*, researchers tested 15 men doing hang cleans—"one of the classic power movements," says study author Gregory Haff, PhD. They used loads between 30 and 90 percent of their one-repetition maximums (the heaviest weight they could lift one time). "The highest power outputs were achieved at about 70 percent of their one-rep max," says Dr. Haff. Stay near that percentage and execute the move in a fast, explosive manner.

WEEK 47 WEEK OF / / TO / / DAY:

STRENGTH TRAINING

		WARMUP SETS			WORK SETS	
EXERCISE	WEIGHT	SET 1 REPS	SET 2 REPS	SET 3 REPS	SET 1 REPS	SET 2 REPS	SET 3 REPS

NOTES:

CARDIO

TYPE	INTENSITY	DURATION

NOTES:

SCULPT AND STRENGTHEN

For healthy ankles and better balance, perform these moves for 30 seconds per leg, three to five times a week.

SINGLE-LEG BALANCE

Stand on one leg for 30 seconds.

SINGLE-LEG DRIBBLE

Dribble a basketball while balancing on one leg.

UNSTABLE BALANCE

Stand on a balance board.

SINGLE-LEG UNSTABLE BALANCE

Stand on a balance board on one leg.

UNSTABLE DRIBBLE

Stand on one leg on a balance board and dribble a basketball.

WEEK 48 | WEEK OF / / TO / / | DAY:

STRENGTH TRAINING

EXERCISE	WEIGHT	WARMUP SETS			WORK SETS		
		SET 1 REPS	SET 2 REPS	SET 3 REPS	SET 1 REPS	SET 2 REPS	SET 3 REPS

NOTES:

CARDIO

TYPE	INTENSITY	DURATION

NOTES:

FUELING UP

ALL-DAY ENERGY

Sentenced to a day of hard labor? Bag the big lunch break. University of Montana researchers found that men work harder and longer when they eat small snacks all day long instead. In the study, wildland firefighters who grazed on small portions of easy-to-eat foods rested less and worked more during a 12-hour shift than when they ate the same number of calories in a large midday meal. Even if you're just cleaning the gutters, well-timed carbohydrate intake is key. "Between 25 and 40 grams an hour provides your muscles with a constant fuel supply," notes study author Brent Ruby, PhD.

FAST FUEL

2 ounces Planters Nut and Chocolate Trail
Mix: 27 grams carbohydrates

Six peanut-butter-cracker sandwiches:
25 grams carbohydrates

16 ounces Gatorade: 28 grams carbohydrates

Clif Builder's Bar: 30 grams carbohydrates

Large apple: 29 grams carbohydrates

WEEK 48 | WEEK OF / / TO / / | DAY:

STRENGTH TRAINING

EXERCISE	WEIGHT	WARMUP SETS			WORK SETS		
		SET 1	SET 2	SET 3	SET 1	SET 2	SET 3
		REPS	REPS	REPS	REPS	REPS	REPS

NOTES: _____

CARDIO

TYPE	INTENSITY	DURATION

NOTES: _____

| WEEK 48 | WEEK OF / / TO / / | DAY: |

CORE POWER

TWICE THE AB WORKOUT

Want a harder core? Then try a harder exercise. Canadian researchers determined that your abs work nearly twice as hard when you do a plank on a Swiss ball instead of on the floor. To perform a plank, get into pushup position but place your forearms on the floor or Swiss ball, then contract your abs and hold. One caveat: "Unless you can hold a plank for 30 seconds, you shouldn't attempt the Swiss-ball version," says Micheal A. Clark, DPT, president of the National Academy of Sports Medicine. That's because trying the advanced exercise before you're ready could strain your back. Pass the test? Do three to five 10-second ball planks, resting on your knees for 2 beats between sets.

STRENGTH TRAINING

EXERCISE	WEIGHT	WARMUP SETS						WORK SETS					
		SET 1		SET 2		SET 3		SET 1		SET 2		SET 3	
			REPS		REPS		REPS		REPS		REPS		REPS

NOTES: _____

CARDIO

TYPE	INTENSITY	DURATION

NOTES: _____

STRETCH IT OUT

TWISTED TRUTH

Stay strong and limber by stretching at the right time. Static stretches—the stretch-and-hold technique you're familiar with—can reduce strength and power when done before your workout, according to a report in the *Strength and Conditioning Journal*. Stretching causes muscle fibers to relax, thus inhibiting the amount of force you're able to produce. Know what to stretch when, for great results.

When you wake up: Stretch your hip flexors, quadriceps, and neck muscles. These muscles are often tight because of the way most men sleep, with their legs bent and shoulders rounded.

Before your workout: Steer clear of static stretches for 1 to 2 hours before you train. Try calisthenics instead.

After you train: Stretch all the muscles used in your workout, and stay consistent—gains in flexibility accrue over time.

In the evening: Before you snooze, stretch your hamstrings, lower back, and glutes. Long hours at your desk tighten these areas.

Hold each stretch for 30 seconds.

WEEK 48   WEEK OF / / TO / /   DAY:

STRENGTH TRAINING

EXERCISE	WEIGHT	WARMUP SETS			WORK SETS		
		SET 1 REPS	SET 2 REPS	SET 3 REPS	SET 1 REPS	SET 2 REPS	SET 3 REPS

NOTES: ___

CARDIO

TYPE	INTENSITY	DURATION

NOTES: ___

SCULPT AND STRENGTHEN

MIX IT UP FOR MUSCLE

The numbers below represent how hard your muscles contract during three lower-body exercises; the higher the number, the greater the effort by that particular muscle.

RECTUS FEMORIS

Stepup: 40
Back squat: 98
Single-leg squat: 15

GLUTEUS MEDIUS

Stepup: 49
Back squat: 31
Single-leg squat: 47

GLUTEUS MAXIMUS

Stepup: 32
Back squat: 34
Single-leg squat: 31

| WEEK 49 | | WEEK OF / / TO / / | | DAY: |

STRENGTH TRAINING

		WARMUP SETS			WORK SETS		
EXERCISE	WEIGHT	SET 1 REPS	SET 2 REPS	SET 3 REPS	SET 1 REPS	SET 2 REPS	SET 3 REPS

NOTES:

CARDIO

TYPE	INTENSITY	DURATION

NOTES:

IRON AID

Lower your golf score in the weight room. Gaining strength can make you a more accurate putter, report researchers at the U.S. Air Force Academy. The study, published in the *Journal of Strength and Conditioning Research*, confirms previous findings that men who weight-train launch the ball farther off the tee. But the researchers also found that men had 30 percent better control on the putting green after an 11-week workout regimen. The golfers performed a mix of classic resistance-training exercises for all their major muscle groups and rotational medicine-ball moves for their core. For instance, they did medicine-ball rotations, medicine-ball throws, Russian twists, and front bridges. Improving your strength, endurance, and flexibility may help your golf swing stay more consistent over the course of 18 holes, the researchers suggest.

WEEK 49 WEEK OF / / TO / / DAY: _____

STRENGTH TRAINING

EXERCISE	WEIGHT	WARMUP SETS SET 1 REPS	WARMUP SETS SET 2 REPS	WARMUP SETS SET 3 REPS	WORK SETS SET 1 REPS	WORK SETS SET 2 REPS	WORK SETS SET 3 REPS

NOTES: _____

CARDIO

TYPE	INTENSITY	DURATION

NOTES: _____

FITNESS FACT
STEEP DECLINE AHEAD

Sure, diet soda is calorie-free carbonation. But if you want a beverage that can actually burn blubber instead of blocking it, drink brewed green tea instead. In fact, green tea may be a more effective fat fighter than previously thought. The credit goes to catechins, chemicals found in varying levels in green tea. In a recent Japanese study, men who drank tea high in catechins lost nearly 5 pounds, compared with no drop in weight for men who drank an ordinary brew. Lead researcher Ichiro Tokimitsu, PhD, suggests that the catechins may help hustle fat molecules out of the bloodstream before they're deposited around your middle. Drink three 15-ounce servings of green tea a day to start losing the lard, he says.

WEEK 49 | **WEEK OF / / TO / /** | **DAY:**

STRENGTH TRAINING

EXERCISE	WEIGHT	WARMUP SETS						WORK SETS					
		SET 1		SET 2		SET 3		SET 1		SET 2		SET 3	
		REPS		REPS		REPS		REPS		REPS		REPS	

NOTES:

CARDIO

TYPE	INTENSITY	DURATION

NOTES:

CORE POWER

DOUBLE CRUNCH

Lie on your back with your feet flat on the floor and a medicine ball between your knees. Rest your hands lightly on your chest. Exhale as you lift your shoulders off the floor and bring your knees to your chest. Grab the ball with your hands and pull it to your chest as you inhale and return your shoulders and legs to the starting position. Transfer the ball back to your legs on the next repetition, and keep alternating ball positions throughout the set. Perform three sets of 12 reps.

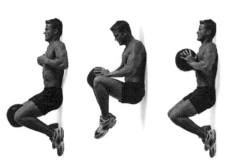

STRENGTH TRAINING

| WEEK 49 | WEEK OF / / TO / / | DAY: |

EXERCISE	WEIGHT	WARMUP SETS						WORK SETS					
		SET 1		SET 2		SET 3		SET 1		SET 2		SET 3	
		REPS		REPS		REPS		REPS		REPS		REPS	

NOTES: _____

CARDIO

TYPE	INTENSITY	DURATION

NOTES: _____

FUELING UP
APPLES FOR ABS

Fruits and vegetables can be muscle foods. In a recent study, Australian researchers found that men who reduced their antioxidant intake by eating just one serving of fruit and two of vegetables daily for 2 weeks felt as if they were exerting more effort than when exercising on a diet rich in antioxidants. Eating several servings of fruit and vegetables daily can make exercise seem easier and help you finish those last reps.

WEEK 50 | WEEK OF / / TO / / | DAY:

STRENGTH TRAINING

EXERCISE	WEIGHT	WARMUP SETS			WORK SETS		
		SET 1 REPS	SET 2 REPS	SET 3 REPS	SET 1 REPS	SET 2 REPS	SET 3 REPS

NOTES:

CARDIO

TYPE	INTENSITY	DURATION

NOTES:

Ask the Trainer

Why do the backs of my knees hurt after 20 minutes on the bike or treadmill?

—Tim, Aurora, CO

Pain in the back of the knee is often caused by something called a Baker's cyst or by an injury of the kneecap. Swelling in the back of the knee is common with a Baker's cyst, but it usually goes away on its own. If it doesn't diminish, you may have injured the meniscal cartilage in the joint, so see a good orthopedic doctor.

| WEEK 50 | WEEK OF / / TO / / | DAY: |

STRENGTH TRAINING

EXERCISE	WEIGHT	WARMUP SETS			WORK SETS		
		SET 1 REPS	SET 2 REPS	SET 3 REPS	SET 1 REPS	SET 2 REPS	SET 3 REPS

NOTES: _____

CARDIO

TYPE	INTENSITY	DURATION

NOTES: _____

WEEK OF / / TO / /   DAY:

STRENGTH TRAINING

EXERCISE	WEIGHT	WARMUP SETS			WORK SETS		
		SET 1 REPS	SET 2 REPS	SET 3 REPS	SET 1 REPS	SET 2 REPS	SET 3 REPS

NOTES:

CARDIO

TYPE	INTENSITY	DURATION

NOTES:

FITNESS FACT

MASTER THE PUSHUP

Another reason to chisel your midsection: Finnish researchers recently discovered that abdominal fat is the best indicator of how many pushups you'll be able to perform, regardless of how much muscle you have. In the study of nearly a thousand men, scientists noted that men with smaller waists fare better in a maximal-pushup test than do men with apparently larger muscles but more abdominal fat. "We found that as waist circumference goes up, performance goes down," notes study author Mikael Fogelholm, DSc. Blame it on gravity, which pulls your bulging belly toward the floor and reduces your mechanical advantage.

Ask the Trainer

Is there an exercise I can do to stop my slouching?
—Kyle, Austin, TX

Begin by stretching your hamstrings and hip flexors. When these muscles are tight, they can cause strain on the lower back. Then try this move from Houston-based personal trainer Carter Hays, CSCS. Do two or three sets of 12 repetitions.

Drop to your hands and knees, arms straight below your shoulders, knees under your hips. Stare between your hands. "Lift your left arm and right leg until they're parallel to the floor. Hold for a count of 4, lower them, and repeat with your opposite arm and leg. That's one repetition.

WEEK 50   WEEK OF / / TO / /   DAY:

STRENGTH TRAINING

EXERCISE	WEIGHT	WARMUP SETS			WORK SETS		
		SET 1 REPS	SET 2 REPS	SET 3 REPS	SET 1 REPS	SET 2 REPS	SET 3 REPS

NOTES: _____

CARDIO

TYPE	INTENSITY	DURATION

NOTES: _____

FUELING UP

JUST SAY YES TO FOOD

A recent Tufts University study found that the less restrictive your diet plan, the greater your chances of long-term weight loss. When researchers randomly assigned 160 people to one of four diets—the Zone, Atkins, Weight Watchers, or Ornish—they found that 50 percent of those following the restrictive Atkins and Ornish approaches had quit after a year, compared with just 35 percent of the people on the more moderate Zone and Weight Watchers plans. But did one erase more weight than the other? No, adherents of both plans netted losses of 10 to 20 pounds. "Each eating strategy reduces caloric intake to a similar extent, so the weight loss is similar," says study author Michael Dansinger, MD. The message: Focus on your ability to grow old with a diet rather than on its gut-busting gimmick.

WEEK 51	WEEK OF / / TO / /	DAY:

STRENGTH TRAINING

EXERCISE	WEIGHT	WARMUP SETS			WORK SETS		
		SET 1 REPS	SET 2 REPS	SET 3 REPS	SET 1 REPS	SET 2 REPS	SET 3 REPS

NOTES:

CARDIO

TYPE	INTENSITY	DURATION

NOTES:

SPOTLIGHT EXERCISE

HANGING SINGLE-KNEE RAISE

Hang from a chinup bar with your palms facing forward and your hands a little farther than shoulder-width apart. Without swinging, raise your left knee as close to your right shoulder as you can, using your abs for power. Tilt your pelvis slightly forward to help. Hold for a second, then return to the starting position. Repeat with your right leg and your left shoulder. Do 8 to 12 repetitions on each side.

WEEK 51 | WEEK OF / / TO / / | DAY:

STRENGTH TRAINING

EXERCISE	WEIGHT	WARMUP SETS						WORK SETS					
		SET 1		SET 2		SET 3		SET 1		SET 2		SET 3	
		REPS	REPS	REPS	REPS	REPS	REPS	REPS	REPS	REPS	REPS	REPS	REPS

NOTES:

CARDIO

TYPE	INTENSITY	DURATION

NOTES:

229

| WEEK 51 | WEEK OF / / TO / / | DAY: |

STRENGTH TRAINING

EXERCISE	WEIGHT	WARMUP SETS			WORK SETS		
		SET 1 REPS	SET 2 REPS	SET 3 REPS	SET 1 REPS	SET 2 REPS	SET 3 REPS

NOTES: _____

CARDIO

TYPE	INTENSITY	DURATION

NOTES: _____

Ask the Trainer

Cycling makes my hips feel tight and inflexible. How can I keep them loose?

—*Jorge, San Antonio, TX*

Cycling causes your pelvis to tilt forward, pulling your glutes out of alignment and forcing you to rely too much on your hamstrings, quadriceps, and lower back. Since your hips act as a brace for your lower back, your back compensates by flexing, extending, and rotating. Release your tight hip flexors and retrain your glutes by performing these lower-body exercises twice a week. For each move, do 10 reps per side.

ACTIVE HIP-FLEXOR STRETCH (SIDE-LYING)

Lie on your left side with your heels near your butt and your knees at waist level. Place your left hand on your left knee. Grab your right ankle, flex your foot toward your knee, then rotate your right leg downward. Pause, return, and repeat for 10 reps. Switch sides.

BACK LUNGE (WITH SIDE BEND)

From a standing position, step back with your left foot and bend your knees 90 degrees. At the same time, reach overhead with your left hand and bend your torso to your right. Then push back up.

FUELING UP

OLIVE OIL

Superpowers: lowers cholesterol, boosts immune system

Secret weapons: monounsaturated fat, vitamin E

Fights against: obesity, cancer, heart disease, high blood pressure

Sidekicks: canola oil, peanut oil, sesame oil

HOW TO USE IT

- Dress up a salad. Making your own salad dressing is only slightly harder than boiling water. Use 1 part olive oil and 2 parts lemon juice, orange juice, vinegar, or wine. Stir them together to blend or just pour each one on the salad.

- Boost flavor. Microwave a couple of tablespoons of oil with red pepper flakes, a crushed garlic clove, or chopped fresh herbs, then filter out the solids with a strainer. Congratulations—you've just made unartificial flavoring. Use it in place of butter.

WEEK 51 | WEEK OF / / TO / / | DAY:

STRENGTH TRAINING

EXERCISE	WEIGHT	WARMUP SETS SET 1 REPS	WARMUP SETS SET 2 REPS	WARMUP SETS SET 3 REPS	WORK SETS SET 1 REPS	WORK SETS SET 2 REPS	WORK SETS SET 3 REPS

NOTES:

CARDIO

TYPE	INTENSITY	DURATION

NOTES:

TRAINING TIP

SIX-PACK MENTALITY

We've said it before: A dog is a great exercise buddy. And now scientists have proved it. Researchers at the University of Victoria in British Columbia found that people who own dogs walk almost twice as much as those who don't have dogs. Credit the dog owners' sense of responsibility and obligation, says study author Ryan Rhodes, PhD. One other key reason: Pets are pushy. Doctors at Northwestern Memorial Hospital in Chicago discovered that when it comes to exercise, dogs are "consistent initiators." So adopting a pooch is like hiring a full-time trainer.

Dog owners exercise, on average, 132 minutes more each week than people who don't own a dog.

WEEK 52	WEEK OF / / TO / /	DAY:

STRENGTH TRAINING

EXERCISE	WEIGHT	WARMUP SETS			WORK SETS		
		SET 1 REPS	SET 2 REPS	SET 3 REPS	SET 1 REPS	SET 2 REPS	SET 3 REPS

NOTES:

CARDIO

TYPE	INTENSITY	DURATION

NOTES:

SPOTLIGHT EXERCISE

STRAIGHT-ARM PULLDOWN

This iron-cross–like exercise brings your arms through 180 degrees of motion against resistance to help built a better back.

Kneel or sit at a high-pulley cable-crossover station, arms to the sides, thumbs up, one handle in each hand.

Pull the handles down and behind your hips so they almost touch your butt. Return slowly to starting position.

WEEK 52 | WEEK OF / / TO / / | DAY:

STRENGTH TRAINING

EXERCISE	WEIGHT	WARMUP SETS			WORK SETS		
		SET 1 REPS	SET 2 REPS	SET 3 REPS	SET 1 REPS	SET 2 REPS	SET 3 REPS

NOTES:

CARDIO

TYPE	INTENSITY	DURATION

NOTES:

WEEK 52 | WEEK OF / / TO / / | DAY:

STRENGTH TRAINING

EXERCISE	WEIGHT	WARMUP SETS			WORK SETS		
		SET 1 REPS	SET 2 REPS	SET 3 REPS	SET 1 REPS	SET 2 REPS	SET 3 REPS

NOTES: _____
_____

CARDIO

TYPE	INTENSITY	DURATION

NOTES: _____
_____

FUELING UP

ARE FORTIFIED FOODS WORTH IT?

Cereal with "extra fiber": A serving of bran cereal already delivers 10 grams; a bowl with "extra fiber" adds 3 more. "It's probably more of a sales gimmick than a health benefit," says Cyndi Thomson, PhD, assistant professor of nutritional sciences at the University of Arizona in Tucson.

Verdict: Good, but not essential

Omega-3-fortified eggs: Omega-3 fatty acids (found mostly in fish oil) may help stave off heart disease, arthritis, even prostate cancer. So these eggs are a nice option, says Dr. Thomson.

Verdict: Crack one open

Calcium-fortified orange juice: A Tufts University study concluded that the body absorbs and uses the calcium in orange juice just as readily as the calcium in milk.

Verdict: Drink up

Enriched bottled water: Even if you drink eight glasses a day, the 10 to 15 percent of the RDAs you get with each serving of B or C vitamin–fortified water isn't excessive, Dr. Thomson says.

Verdict: Not worth the money

Ask the Trainer

Are there any protein powders that aren't high in cholesterol?

—Max, Brooklyn, NY

Soy has none, whey has some, but the mixes are mostly benign because neither one will cause cholesterol buildup in your veins. It's saturated fat you should worry about—in the mix and in your mixer. Look for a protein mix with less than 1 gram of saturated fat, and use skim milk instead of whole, which adds 4.5 grams for every 8 ounces.

| WEEK 52 | WEEK OF / / TO / / | DAY: |

STRENGTH TRAINING

EXERCISE	WEIGHT	WARMUP SETS SET 1 REPS	WARMUP SETS SET 2 REPS	WARMUP SETS SET 3 REPS	WORK SETS SET 1 REPS	WORK SETS SET 2 REPS	WORK SETS SET 3 REPS

NOTES:

CARDIO

TYPE	INTENSITY	DURATION

NOTES:

NOW WHAT?

Congratulations! You have completed a year's worth of training workouts. Now is the time to reflect on your accomplishments and take steps to make sure you stick to the good habits you've formed over the past 52 weeks.

It's also the time to think about what you'll do next—and how to keep it fresh. We should have a "refresh" button for everything: a bitter co-worker, a lame bar scene, the National Hockey League. Just a click or two could give us instant improvement.

Same with tired workouts. Maybe yours has frozen up like a gym version of Windows 95. You may think you have to reboot, or even upgrade. Instead, all you need are a few tweaks for a faster, more enjoyable, more effective workout.

Take a typical guy's stale routine: treadmill for 5 minutes, then bench presses until someone asks if he's almost done—in which case he's suddenly on his last set. Next, a few rows, curls, and crunches, then a quick toe touch and he's out.

You can do better, beginning with your warmup. "Most men warm up with a few minutes of light cycling or jogging," says Brad Jordan, NASM CPT, a personal trainer in Dayton, Ohio. And that's fine if all you plan to do in your workout is lower-body exercise. But an upper-body workout demands something that's more in sync with your plans. "Switch your warmup to jumping rope, rowing lightly, or using any cardio machine, like an elliptical trainer, that makes you pump your arms," Jordan says.

As for the rest of your routine . . . stop calling it routine. Refresh it, and yourself, with these moves.

Start with your hamstrings. "Most men do the exercises they like first and save the ones they know they hate for last," says Steve Lischin, NASM-CPT. "Toward the end of a workout, they either put little effort into these exercises or just skip them entirely." Performing your workout in the opposite order can give muscles you tend to overlook (such as your hamstrings) the attention they deserve. And saving your favorites for last can help you recharge when your energy level is in decline.

Stretch between sets. "Don't stretch only when your muscles feel tight," says Jordan. Stretching the muscles you're working not only helps them stay loose, but can also increase your range of motion, allowing you to work more muscle fibers with each additional set.

Take a coffee break. Anytime you draw your legs toward your midsection—reverse crunches, V-ups—you emphasize the lower portion of your abs. These moves also stress your hip flexors, the muscles on the front of your thighs. When these muscles are involved, your abs exert less than full effort, and you end up with tight hip flexors.

Overcome this tendency by pretending there's a cup of coffee resting just below your belly button. Before bringing your legs up each time, imagine tilting that cup toward your legs first. "This redirects your body positioning, so the effort stays concentrated on the lower abs," says Len Kravitz, PhD, coordinator of exercise science at the University of New Mexico in Albuquerque.

Close your eyes while exercising. This helps you visualize the muscles you're working, which is especially helpful for posterior muscle groups like your back, hamstrings, and butt. (Exceptions allowed when that brunette happens by.) Also try closing your eyes during any exercise that involves balance, such as a one-legged squat. "It challenges the neuromuscular system and helps you establish better balance," says Carter Hays, CSCS, a Houston-based personal trainer. "It's actually harder closing just one eye than both eyes; it's weird."

Change your inclination. Rather than do three sets of dumbbell presses followed by three sets of incline presses, combine the two exercises. Start with one set of chest presses on a flat bench. Then raise the bench one notch from the flat position—to about 15 to 20 degrees—for your second set. Continue raising the angle one notch per set, stopping at the notch before vertical. "This lets you exhaust more muscle fibers by working your chest through five or six different angles instead of just the basic two," says Wayne Westcott, CSCS, PhD, a Massachusetts-based exercise researcher. You'll actually end up doing fewer sets, so you'll save time, too.

Get twisted. During the standard single-arm dumbbell row, your palm faces in as you raise and lower the weight along the side of your chest. To get more out of the move, rotate your wrist inward 180 degrees as you lower the dumbbell so that your thumb ends up pointing behind you when your arm is completely straight. This rotation helps adduct the scapula, working the back through a fuller range of motion for added strength and size.

Stop and go. Instead of raising and lowering the weight in one continuous motion, pause for a second about halfway up, continue the movement, and then pause again about halfway down. "In a set of 8 to 12 repetitions, you'll add only an extra 16 to 24 seconds to each set, but you'll be able to exhaust your muscles faster using less weight," says Lischir. This tactic works great with shoulder presses, lateral raises, and bent-over lateral raises.

Lower the weight with one leg. Your muscles are much stronger during the eccentric phase of an exercise—when the weight is being lowered. With leg presses, leg curls, and leg extensions, consider the "two up, one down" option. Try pressing or curling the weight up with both legs, then slowly lowering the weight back down using only one leg. This lets you work your muscles even harder in the same amount of time without constantly needing to change the weight, says Dr. Westcott.

Spread 'em. Change your hand spacing with each set of barbell curls, instead of keeping them placed at shoulder width for all your repetitions. "Spreading your hands a few inches farther out stresses more of the inner portion of your biceps, while bringing your hands in a few inches builds more of the outer part," says Lischin. Or, try switching from the standard shoulder-width grip on a barbell to an angled position with an EZ-curl bar.

Run the rack. Save time on the last dumbbell exercise in your workout. Instead of doing three sets of shoulder presses, biceps curls, or any dumbbell move, start with a weight that's about 50 percent of what you usually use to do 10 to 12 repetitions. Perform the exercise six times, then quickly grab the weight that's one increment heavier. Continue working your way up in weight until you finally find one that you can't lift six times using proper technique. Then reverse this process by grabbing a slightly lighter weight and completing as many repetitions as possible, even if you can manage only a few. Keep moving down the rack until you're left using the lightest set of dumbbells possible.

PHOTO CREDITS

© Rodale Images: 17, 18, 94

© Beth Bischoff: 30, 41, 43, 44, 49, 52, 53, 61, 73, 86, 89, 98, 104, 108, 113, 131, 136, 147, 148, 172, 181, 186, 195, 200, 210, 223, 227, 229, 233

© Kagan Mcleod: 32, 34, 37, 57, 69, 103, 116, 120, 125, 134, 141, 159, 160, 165, 177, 212

© Chris Philpot: 64

© Mika-Zefa/Corbis: 76

© IT Stock Free/PictureQuest: 80

© Jamie Grill/Age Fotostock: 152

© Friedemann Vogel/Bongarts/Getty Images: 169

© Melissa Punch: 190, 196

ALSO AVAILABLE FROM RODALE BOOKS . . .

MensHealth®

MEN'S HEALTH®
ULTIMATE DUMBELL GUIDE
By Myatt Murphy

This indispensable guide features a comprehensive list of dumbbell moves that can be combined into more than 21,000 innovative exercises, plus instructions for creating millions of your own personalized combination moves.

MEN'S HEALTH®
HOME WORKOUT BIBLE
By Lou Schuler and Michael Mejia

From custom training plans to equipment buying advice, *Men's Health® Home Workout Bible* provides complete guidelines for turning your home into a state-of-the-art fitness center.

MEN'S HEALTH®
THE BODY YOU WANT IN THE TIME YOU HAVE
By Myatt Murphy

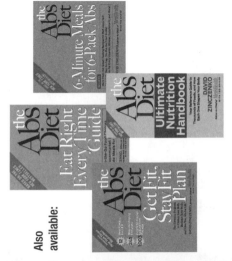

Organized by how many days a week and minutes a day you have to exercise, *Men's Health® The Body Your Want in the Time You Have* offers 120 workouts to burn fat, build muscle, and stay fit—no matter how much (or little) time you have!

MEN'S HEALTH®
POWER TRAINING
By Robert dos Remedios, MA, CSCS

Optimize your muscle and strength gains while speeding fat loss with *Men's Health® Power Training*'s short, intense training sessions, flexible workout plans, and total-body exercises.

MEN'S HEALTH®
HARD BODY PLAN
By Larry Keller and
the editors of *Men's Health*®

Men's Health® Hard Body Plan gives you three cutting-edge 12-week full-body muscle plans for bigger shoulders, bulging biceps, ripped abs, a leaner torso, and strong legs in just 12 weeks!

MEN'S HEALTH®
GYM BIBLE
By Michael Mejia and
Myatt Murphy

Whether you're a novice or just looking to get more from your workouts, *Men's Health® Gym Bible* offers comprehensive information on everything from negotiating gym memberships to proper machine techniques.

THE ABS DIET
By David Zinczenko

Want to strip away belly fat and have beach-ready abs all year? Let *Men's Health* editor-in-chief David Zinczenko teach you how with the *New York Times* best-selling *Abs Diet* series.

Also available:

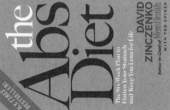